Sleeping Disorder Explained

The Ultimate Guide about Sleeping Disorders

Sleeping Disorders Overview, Types, Treatments, Causes, Symptoms, Other Complications, Future Treatments, Alternative Medicines, and much more included!

By: Frederick Earlstein

Foreword

One of the most interesting things about humans is that around 1/3 of our lives consist of sleep! Sleep patterns vary from one individual to another but on average, an adult person should at least have 7 to 8 hours of sleep per day.

Up to now, scientists and researchers haven't fully scratched the surface yet on why it is necessary for humans to sleep. They also haven't fully understood yet the mechanisms of why the act of sleeping helps us recharge and restore both our physical and mental aspects.

According to medical experts if our sleep is frequently disrupted it will most certainly affect our health because it can be a cause of fatigue. Fatigue can eventually affect one's performance and also cause other significant physical, mental, and even social disturbances.

Unfortunately, the cases of sleep disorders especially among adult Americans are continuously rising. Approximately around 75% of Americans, and 30% of children are diagnosed with various sleep disorder/ disturbance conditions, or they are frequently experiencing symptoms of it most nights in a week.

Losing sleep or not having enough sleep is detrimental to one's health. According to medical experts, it can eventually affect one's life and organs in the body which can progress into serious illnesses.

Fortunately, medical practitioners, schools, and other wellness institutions are now educating the people about the benefits of having enough sleep, and the treatments available to overcome various sleeping disorders. You don't need to suffer sleepless nights anymore if you follow your doctor's advice, and find ways on how you can improve your condition.

This book will guide you about everything you need to know regarding the sleep disorder condition. We will discuss the overview, the various types of sleeping disorders, the causes, and symptoms. We will also provide you relevant information on how you can treat your disorders, the alternative medicine or therapies available as well as the future of sleep disorder treatment.

Table of Contents

Introduction 1

  Development of the Field of Sleep 2

  Non – Rapid Eye Movement 4

    Stage 1 Non – Rapid Eye Movement 4

    Stage 2 Non – Rapid Eye Movement 5

    Stage 3 and Stage 4 Non – Rapid Eye Movement 5

  Rapid Eye Movement (REM) 5

Chapter One: What is Insomnia? 7

  Classifications of Insomnia 8

  Classification of Chronic Insomnia 9

    Psychological Insomnia 10

    Idiopathic Insomnia 10

    Paradoxical Insomnia 11

  Sleep Hygiene 12

  Causes of Insomnia 13

    Insomnia Caused by Mental Disorder/s 14

    Insomnia Caused by Medical Condition 14

    Insomnia Caused by Drugs, Medications, and Other Substances 15

  Other Causes of Insomnia 16

    Limit – Setting Disorder 16

Short – Term Insomnia Disorder 17

Treating Insomnia 18

Chapter Two: Sleep – Related Breathing Disorders.............. 21

Obstructive Sleep Apnea (in Adults) 22

Obstructive Sleep Apnea (in Children)............................. 23

Central Sleep Apnea Syndromes 24

Central Sleep Apnea with Cheyne – Stokes Breathing. 24

Central Sleep Apnea Caused by Medical Disorders
without Cheyne – Stokes Breathing 25

Central Sleep Apnea Caused by High – Altitude
Periodic Breathing... 25

Central Sleep Apnea Caused by Medication Intake 26

Primary Central Sleep Apnea (in Infants) 26

Primary Central Sleep Apnea in Premature Infants 26

Treatment Emergent Central Sleep Apnea..................... 27

Sleep – Related Hypoventilation Disorders 27

Obesity Hypoventilation Syndrome 27

Congenital Central Alveolar Hypoventilation Syndrome
.... 28

Late – Onset Central Hypoventilation with
Hypothalamic Dysfunction 28

Idiopathic Central Alveolar Hypoventilation............... 29

Sleep – Related Hypoventilation Caused by Substance or Medications 29

Sleep – Related Hypoventilation Caused by Medical Disorder 29

Isolated Symptoms 30

Snoring 30

Catathrenia 31

Chapter Three: Central Disorders of Hypersomnolence & Circadian Rhythm Sleep – Wake Disorders 33

Central Disorders of Hypersomnolence 34

Narcolepsy Type I 34

Causes of Narcolepsy 38

Diagnosing Narcolepsy 39

Treating Narcolepsy 40

Narcolepsy Type II 41

Idiopathic Hypersomnia 42

Kleine – Levin Syndrome 42

Causes of Hypersomnia 43

Hypersomnia Caused by Medical Disorders 43

Hypersomnia Caused by Substances or Medicine in - Take 43

Hypersomnia with Psychiatric Disorder 43

Insufficient Sleep Syndrome 44

Circadian Rhythm Sleep – Wake Disorders........................ 45

Delayed Sleep – Wake Phase Disorder 45

Advanced Sleep – Wake Phase Disorder......................... 46

Irregular Sleep – Wake Rhythm Disorder 46

Non – 24 Hour Sleep – Wake Rhythm Sleep Disorder . 47

Shift Work Disorder.. 47

Jet Lag Disorder.. 48

Circadian Rhythm Sleep Disorder Not Otherwise
Specified 48

Chapter Four: Parasomnias 51

Disorders of Arousal from Non – Rapid Eye Movement
Sleep 52

Confusional Arousals 52

Sleep Walking.. 53

Sleep Terrors 54

Sleep – Related Eating Disorder 54

Recurrent Isolated Sleep Paralysis............................ 55

Nightmare Disorder.. 55

Other Types of Parasomnias 56

Exploding Head Syndrome 56

Sleep – Related Hallucinations............................. 57

Sleep Enuresis.. 58

Causes of Parasomnias 58

Parasomnias Caused by Medical Disorder 58

Parasomnias Caused by Medication in – take or Other
Substances 59

Sleep Talking 59

Chapter Five: Sleep – Related Movement Disorders 61

Restless Legs Syndrome.. 62

Periodic Limb Movement Disorder................................. 64

Sleep – Related Leg Cramps 65

Sleep – Related Bruxism.. 65

Sleep – Related Rhythmic Movement Disorder 66

Benign Sleep Myoclonus of Infancy 67

Propriospinal Myoclonus at Sleep Onset 68

Causes of Sleep – Related Movement Disorder................. 68

Sleep – Related Movement Disorder Caused by a
Medical Disorder.. 68

Sleep – Related Movement Disorder Caused by a
Medication in – Take or Substance 69

Isolated Symptoms of Sleep – Related Movement Disorder
.... 69

Excessive Fragmentary Myoclonus 69

Hypnagogic Foot Tremor (HFT) and Alternating Muscle
Activation (ALMA)... 70

Hypnic Jerks or Sleep Starts 70

Other Type of Sleeping Disorders 71

Environmental Sleep Disorder 71

Chapter Six: Alternative Medicine and Herbal Remedies ... 73

Conventional Treatments vs. Unconventional Treatments
.... 74

Psychological Treatment 74

Pharmacological Treatment 75

Limitation in Drug Therapies 76

Alternative Therapies 77

Herbal Remedies for Sleep Disorders 78

Medicinal Herbs as Remedies 80

Ginseng 82

Kava Kava (Piper methysticum) 83

Passion flower (Passiflora incarnata) 84

Hops (Humulus lupulus) 85

Physiological Alternative Treatments 86

Melatonin 86

L – Tryptophan and 5 – Hydroxytryptophan 87

Other Alternative Approach 88

Acupuncture 88

Low Energy Emission Therapy (LEET) 89

FAQs in taking Herbal Medicines to Treat Sleeping Disorders 90

Conclusion 97

Chapter Seven: The Future of Sleep Disorder Treatments .. 99

The Future of Conducting Sleep Disorder Treatments .. 100

At – Home Sleep Testing Devices................................. 100

Phone Apps and Wearable Technology 102

Telehealth.. 103

Further Research about Sleeping Disorders.................... 103

Chapter Summary... 105

Photo Credits 121

References 123

Introduction

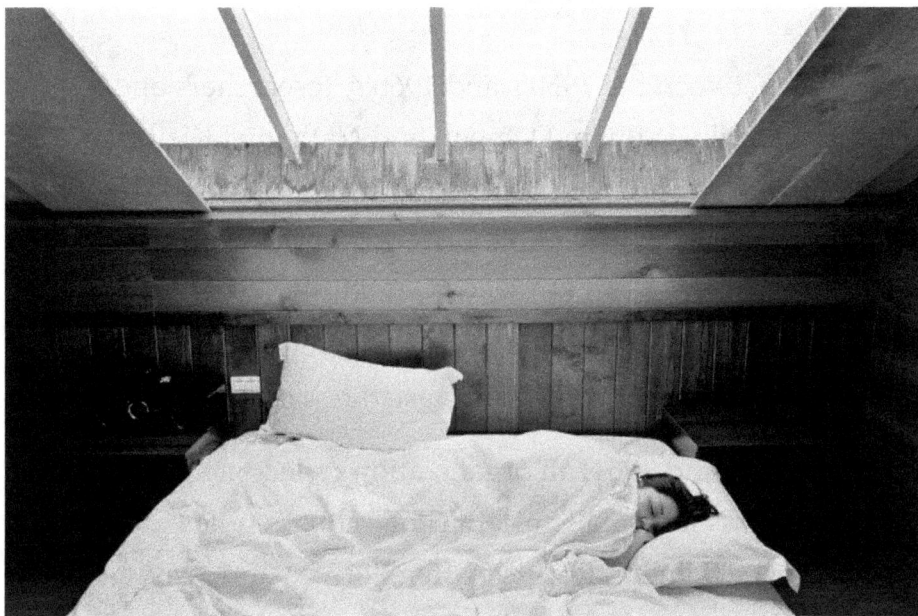

Ever since the beginning of time, humans are very fascinated and curious about the nature of sleep. For instance, around 1836, famous novelist Charles Dickens, published a series of works called the "Posthumous Papers of the Pickwick Club" wherein he described a boy who is obese, and someone who snored loudly and heavily. This is where a term of sleep disorder called Pickwickian Syndrome was coined but it is now known today as Obesity Hypoventilation Syndrome (OHS). This chapter will give you a brief history of how the field of sleep/ sleep disorder has been established, and also a brief introduction about the most common form of sleep disorder in the world.

Development of the Field of Sleep

Between the 1950's and 1960's, researchers and scientists like William Dement, and Nathaniel Kleitman pioneered studies about sleep and its various disorders as well as sleep stages and patterns. And through the advent of technology, it paved the way for medical practitioners to learn more about the field and also developed treatments and therapies that could help ease the symptoms.

Around 1961, an organization called Sleep Research Society was informally established with pioneers including Kleitman, Dement, Rechtschaffen, Jouvet, and Aserinsky. In 1968, Doctor Anthony Kales and Allan Rechtschaffen have authored a book called "A Manual of Standardized Technology Techniques and Scoring Systems for Sleep Stages of Human Subjects" which is still being used today.

Around 1975, an organization called the Association of Sleep Disorders Centers or ASDC was established, it is now known today as AASM or American Academy of Sleep Medicine.

In 1990's, other sleep societies and research organizations had been developed like the CSS or Clinical Sleep Society, APSS or Association of Professional Sleep Societies, ABSM or the American Board of Sleep Medicine, and the NSF or the National Sleep Foundation. Within the same year, AASM was able to develop the 1st edition of ICSD or International Classification of Sleep Disorders which describes various types of sleep disorders known today. A 2nd edition of the same title was published in 2005, and has been updated ever since.

Insomnia is perhaps the most common type of sleep disorder and is being experienced by people all over the world. For instance, in the U.S. alone, the cost of treatment for the disorder as well as the loss productivity and damages because of insomnia – related incidents exceeds around $00 billion annually. Insomnia can be described as difficulty falling and maintaining asleep but for most people, perhaps it's simply another form of restlessness. Around 30% of adults suffer from insomnia for a year or so. It is classified as mostly chronic or severe, primary or secondary, and sometimes a combination of both. Insomnia may also progress to other complications like anxiety and depression. It also occurs mostly to women, and comes with aging as well.

Unfortunately, insomnia is not the only form of sleep disorder. There are various types of it which you will thoroughly learn in the next few chapters. The following are the other classifications of sleep disorders:

- Sleep – Related Breathing Disorders
    - o Obstructive Sleep Apnea Disorders
    - o Central Sleep Apnea Syndrome
    - o Sleep – Related Hypoventilation Disorder
- Central Disorders of Hyper - somnolence
- Circadian Rhythm Sleep – Wake Disorders
- Parasomnias
    - o NREM – Related Parasomnias
    - o REM – Related Parasomnias
    - o Other types
- Sleep – Related Movement Disorders

Non – Rapid Eye Movement

Stage 1 Non – Rapid Eye Movement

The stage 1of non – rapid eye movement sleep usually represents very slight sleep where a patient can be easily aroused or disrupted. When it comes to the EEG pattern of NREM sleep stage 1, it has mixed frequency pattern and also low voltage.

Stage 2 Non – Rapid Eye Movement

The NREM sleep stage 2 is characterized as steep spindles and appears as K – complexes on the EEG. A typical night of sleep occurs mostly in Stage 2 NREM sleep.

Stage 3 and Stage 4 Non – Rapid Eye Movement

Collectively, stage 3 and 4 NREM sleep are referred to as slow wave sleep or delta slepp.

Rapid Eye Movement (REM)

The REM sleep also consists of mixed frequency activity in the EEG with a relatively low voltage. It is also somewhat the same with wakefulness or stage 1 but with the appearance of episodic REM. The main characteristic of a REM sleep is a low level of muscle tone.

Chapter One: What is Insomnia?

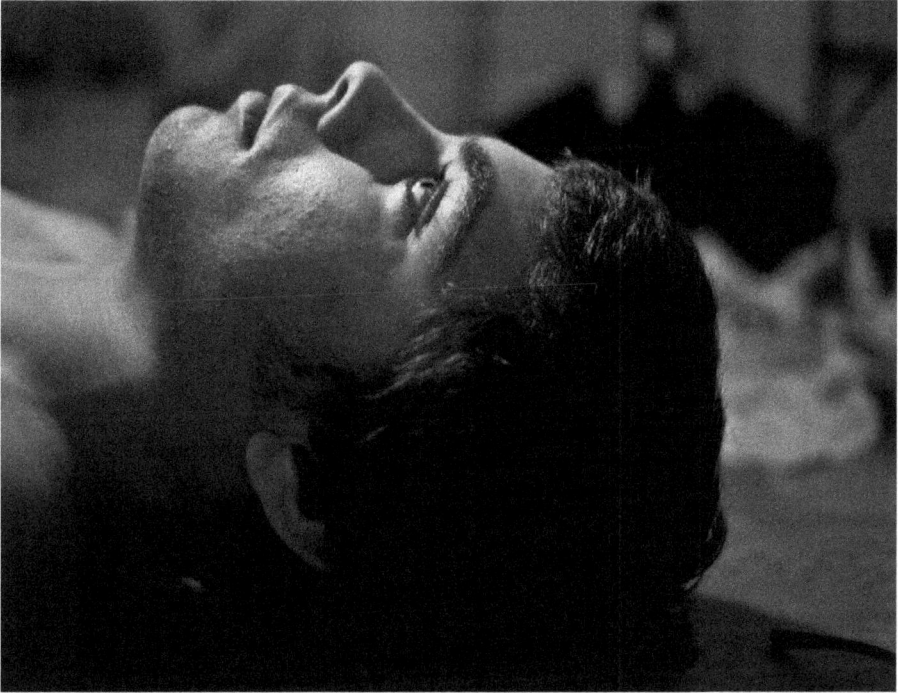

Insomnia is a type of sleep disorder that's being experienced by around 50% of adults in the world. 1 in 10 experiences chronic insomnia and it is twice as common in older people as well as women. It's the common term used when people are having a hard time falling asleep, staying asleep, and even waking up in the morning. It's the lack of experiencing a restorative sleep that gets a normal person going to start the day. This disorder can be classified into two; primary or secondary, and acute or chronic. This chapter will give you a wealth of information about the different classifications, its causes, common symptoms, diagnosis, complications, and possible treatments.

Classifications of Insomnia

Insomnia results to some form of daytime impairment. It can be classified as primary insomnia, secondary insomnia, chronic insomnia, and acute insomnia.

Primary Insomnia

This is a form of insomnia that is mostly attributed to psychological conditioning processes, and not so much to environmental or medical causes.

Secondary Insomnia

This is a form of insomnia that is attributed to psychiatric, external and medical causes. Doctors usually treat the underlying disorders of this condition.

Acute Insomnia vs. Chronic Insomnia

Once the doctor has identified the classification (i.e. primary or secondary), the next step is to determine whether it is an acute insomnia or a chronic one. Acute insomnia is usually caused by stress in life and emotional or physical discomforts. It can also be caused by constantly taking harmful substances like drugs, alcohol, steroids, too much caffeine intake etc., which can condition a person to have sleepless nights, and can also be detrimental to one's health. On the other hand, chronic insomnia is caused by various medical and external factors that can pose treatment challenges to both the doctors and patients. Chronic insomnia is the most common form of the disorder, and can be classified into sub – types which will be discussed in the next section below.

Classification of Chronic Insomnia

Chronic insomnia is classified into different sub – types including the following:

- Psychological Insomnia
- Idiopathic Insomnia
- Paradoxical Insomnia

Psychological Insomnia

Among the 3 sub – types aforementioned, this one is the most prevalent in patients. This is a kind of chronic insomnia that usually lasts for about a month, and it's not caused by external factors. Rather, it is caused by a learned response that teaches one's body to not fall asleep when a person plans to fall asleep. If you happen to have this, it means that you can easily fall asleep when you don't "plan" for it but when you do plan to sleep on normal bedtime or naps, sleep onset is hard to do.

Idiopathic Insomnia

This type of chronic insomnia is also known as "life – long insomnia." It is perhaps one of the most detrimental cases because it can already occur at a very young age usually early childhood or even at the infancy stage, and progresses into adulthood. According to medical experts, there seems to be no external factors affecting this condition, and no other forms of sleeping disorder can caused one to have an idiopathic insomnia.

Paradoxical Insomnia

This is formerly known as "Sleep State Misperception." The termed 'paradoxical or misperception' is coined because this chronic form of insomnia is one where a patient complaints about experiencing insomnia without any actual evidence or symptom if the disorder. Patients usually complains of being awake all night when in fact through the help of EEGs or Electroencephalograms, sleep was achieved. Sometimes patients also have had a normal sleep but still complain that he/she didn't get any at all. It's like you already get enough sleep but still felt restless in the morning.

Usually, the treatment or therapy being done is to write in the so – called 'sleep diary' where the patient should record their sleeping habits over a certain period of time (1 week to about a month). This is done so that the patient can see the irregularities in their own sleeping habits, and how it affects their bedtime schedules or daytime naps. Doctors will then point out the inconsistencies through the sleep diary so that they can both identify the misperception of sleep.

Sleep Hygiene

Sleep hygiene is a term that refers to a healthy sleeping habit. On the other hand, there's also a medical term called Inadequate Sleeping Hygiene which is a set of bad habits that usually causes a patient to sleep poorly. Generally speaking, insomnia is caused by poor sleeping habits which is why there are certain sleep hygiene practices and guidelines that patients suffering from insomnia or other sleep disorders should follow so that they can maintain being asleep longer and allow the body to use that time to recharge, and restore organ functions. Following the tips below will dramatically improve your ability to fall and maintain asleep:

Tip #1: Follow a waking and sleeping routine. A patient should get up at the same time or sleep at the same time every day.

Tip #2: Go to your bed only when you're tired.

Tip #3: Create a relaxing 'pre – sleep rituals'

Tip #4: Eat a healthy and balanced diet.

Tip #5: Exercise regularly.

Tip #6: Never perform extreme exercises at least 4 hours before your bedtime.

Tip #7: Maintain a regular routine or sleeping schedule.

Tip #8: Avoid caffeine in – take at least 6 hours before bedtime

Tip #9: As much as possible avoid drinking alcohol or too much of it.

Tip #10: Do not smoke

Tip #11: If you need to nap, then do it at the same time every day

Tip #12: If you need to use sleeping pills then make sure that you follow your doctor's advice.

Tip #13: Use your bed for sleeping purposes only, and avoid doing other activities in it like studying, working, watching TV, reading etc.

Tip #14: Make your bed a clean and relaxing space

Tip #15: Whenever you're going to sleep, you should block out the noise and the light inside the room.

Causes of Insomnia

Insomnia can be due to several causes including a mental disorder, medical condition, and constant exposure to drugs or other substances. This section will provide you a wealth of information on why such things can cause acute or chronic insomnia.

Insomnia Caused by Mental Disorder/s

As the name suggests, this is a form of insomnia that is mainly caused by a mental illness. It usually occurs for about a month, and it's mostly related to patients that have also been diagnosed with depression or anxiety disorders. The main challenge for doctors when it comes to treating the underlying cause is to determine if the mental disorder is causing the insomnia or another form of sleeping disorder is causing the mental illness. For instance, a patient experiencing chronic forms of insomnia may feel depress as a result of difficulty in sleeping. Alternately, one who feels depress or anxious can also experience insomnia as a symptom.

Insomnia Caused by Medical Condition

There are a lot of medical conditions that can potentially cause short – term or chronic insomnia. Some of the most common medical conditions usually include those that bring about so much pain (physically and emotionally) or discomfort. Such kind of insomnia is more common among the elderly but can also happen in any age.

Insomnia Caused by Drugs, Medications, and Other Substances

Another form of insomnia is caused by drug or alcohol abuse, and/or the withdrawal of it. Such substances often include sedatives, opiates, alcohol, hypnotic drugs, and stimulants. Substances like these can greatly disturb one's sleep pattern one way or another. The effect can great vary depending on how much of these substances were ingested, they type of substance used, the duration, and other extrinsic/ intrinsic factors. For instance, regular alcohol intake can reduce one's sleep latency, wakefulness, REM or rapid eye movement which is something that is needed during sleep. Alcohol intake can also produce sleep fragmentation, and likelihood of nightmares can often occur due to reduced REM. Drug substances on the other hand can increase respiratory problems as these drugs relax the muscles which can provide an obstruction in the upper airway.

Sometimes medications can also have insomnia or other sleep disorders as a side – effect including Beta – Blockers, Thiazides, Corticosteroids, Decongestants, Calcium blockers, Adrenocorticotropic Hormones, Anti – metabolites,

Monoamine Oxidase Inhibitors, Oral Contraceptives, Stimulants, Thyroid Hormones, Bronchodilators to name a few.

Other Causes of Insomnia

There other lesser known types of insomnia such as the Behavioral Insomnia or Limit – Setting Disorder which mostly occurs in children and babies as well as Short – Term Insomnia Disorder.

Limit – Setting Disorder

This is also known as Behavioral Insomnia, and it's a type of insomnia that occurs in infants and kids. Aside from the sleeping tips mentioned above, parents should also make sure that they practice sleeping hygiene on their children so that they can maintain this kind of habit and not have trouble sleeping.

If your child has been diagnosed with behavioral insomnia, then ensure that you don't put toys or other sort of distractions (especially for infants) during bedtime. You also don't want to let your child get used to having you around like falling asleep in your arms or leave them with their bottles because these habits will make them dependent on external factors to initiate sleep. They'd be better off in sleeping naturally on their own and not depend on anything; it's sometimes necessary but shouldn't be practiced on a regular basis. As a parent, you should create a healthy bedtime schedule or routine for your child like reading them stories or something like that.

Short – Term Insomnia Disorder

This is also referred to as Adjustment Insomnia, and it is quite common in today's high – stress and fast – paced culture. A lot of people experience a short – term insomnia wherein one finds it difficult to initiate or maintain sleep for a couple of days or at some point in time. External factors can cause short – term insomnia such as stress, anticipation, illness, excitement, changing schedules, time zones, pain due to loss of someone or something, reactions to certain medications, marital problems, financial, work or family problems etc. It's very common especially for people going through tough times but since it's only temporary, it typically corrects itself once the stressor is gone or alleviated

Treating Insomnia

According to medical practitioners, insomnia is usually a secondary condition, and in most cases it's only treated once the primary condition or other medical condition is naturally cured. For instance, if a patient suffers from arthritis and experiences extreme pain, he/she will most likely experience sleepless nights, and be given a pain – reliever so that he/she can properly sleep.

When it comes to insomnia being the primary condition, the doctor will of course treat it independently. They will suggest their patients to go to the so – called insomnia clinic which is more of like a sleeping laboratory where doctors will use various therapeutic methods and apply such techniques to help their patients. Such therapies include the following:

- **Group Therapy:** This is usually applied to patients if the doctor would like to know other possible underlying psychological causes of a patient's insomnia, and so that the patient themselves can hear the causes of other people's insomnias.

- **Light Therapy:** This method helps the patient to adjust their circadian rhythm or body rhythm so that they can have the ability to sleep at proper times.

- **Self – Control Technique:** This is a technique where are trained to control their psychological parameters to gain control over their ability to sleep. It's also a helpful method for patients who may feel like their lives are in chaos for various reasons.

- **Biofeedback:** This is a technique where patients are trained to control their physiological parameters to also gain control over their insomnia. Such parameters include muscle tension, EEGs, and skin temperature.

- **Sleep Restriction:** This is a technique that's commonly applied for older patients suffering from chronic insomnia. It's also perfect for people who tend to stay up late at night but only sleep for a couple of hours, and not the recommended the 7 to 8 hours per day.

- **Sleep Hygiene guidelines:** This is what we've previously mentioned in previous sections. This is where sleeping diary comes in handy.

Chapter Two: Sleep – Related Breathing Disorders

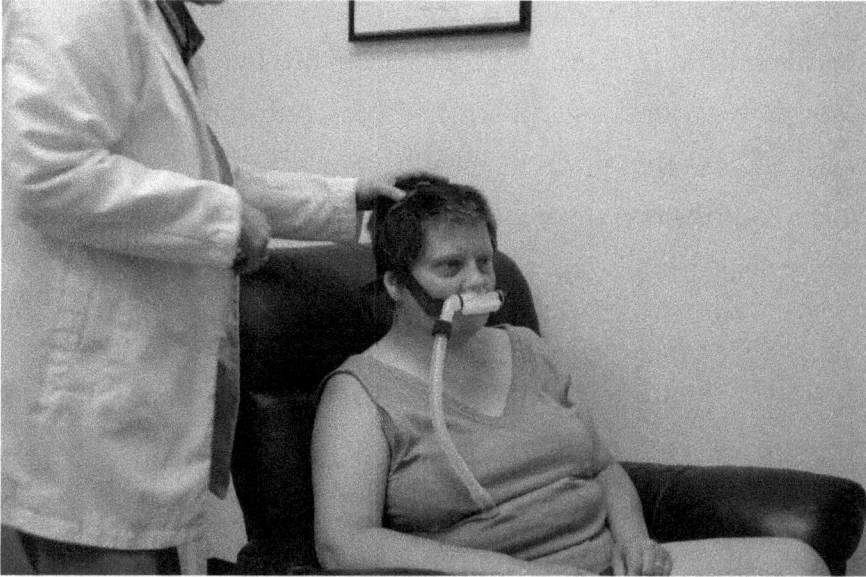

The next most common form of sleep disorder is classified as sleep – related breathing disorders. It is divided into two which is those caused by the central origin, and caused by a form of obstruction. Central breathing disorders are usually described as the lack of the lungs effort due to central nervous disorder or heart dysfunction. On the other hand, sleep – related breathing disorders due to obstructive respiratory is usually associated with various forms of body obstructions such as obesity, inflamed tissues in the upper airways, or large tonsils and tongue. This chapter will provide you with a lot of information about the various types and classifications of sleep – related breathing disorders.

Obstructive Sleep Apnea (in Adults)

Obstructive Sleep Apnea is one of the most common sleep – related breathing disorders next to insomnia. It is also quite dangerous and affects both adults and kids but the good news is that it can be easy to diagnosed and treated. This form of sleep disorder happens when the presence of hypopneas and obstructive apneas are repeated.

An apnea is a respiratory event with a cessation of airflow in the lungs or airways for around 10 seconds, and classified as continued respiratory effort. On the other hand, hypopnea is the decrease of airflow in the lungs which is reduced to around 30% or more in amplitude. Apnea and hypopnea are usually linked with oxygen desaturation. Oxygen desaturation is where hemoglobin in the blood is saturated by oxygen in a reduced amount. Both apnea and hypopnea are also linked with other body events like snoring, body jerks, limb movements, and EEG arousals, and these are usually the symptoms that a patient experiences.

Obstructive Sleep Apnea (OSA) are known to be a contributing factor in other serious types of illnesses like heart diseases, high blood pressure, depression, EDS or excessive daytime sleepiness, morning headaches, loss of memory and concentration, and stroke just to name a few.

Being overweight or diagnosed as obese is one of the main reasons also why patients suffer from OSA. Usually those people with large neck circumferences and excess body fats are at higher risk in being diagnosed with the disorder, and males who are around 30 years old and above are affected by this.

OSA can be diagnosed with the help of AHI or Apnea Hypopnea Index, and RDI or Respiratory Disturbance Index.

Obstructive Sleep Apnea (in Children)

Just like how it is in adults, children experiencing obstructive sleep apnea or hypopneas also have any of the following symptoms including headaches upon waking up, snoring, oxygen desaturation, hypercapnia, and difficulty in breathing or labored breathing. Sometimes paradoxical respiratory effort in the child's rib cage can also be experienced. The main demographic affected by OSA in babies or children are those who are also obese/ overweight and also those who have Down's syndrome. Mild cases of OSA in children can be severe and long – lasting, and it can also affect their physical and mental growth. Medical experts believe that it's also one of the causes of SIDS or Sudden Infant Death Syndrome; an event where a baby dies during their sleep without any sort of symptom or warning.

The main causes of obstructive apnea or hypopnea in kids could be big tonsils or adenoids. The usual treatment given is called a tonsillectomy/ adenoidectomy as well as CPAP or Continuous Positive Airway Pressure.

Central Sleep Apnea Syndromes

There are several types of Central Sleep Apnea Syndrome which we will discuss here. CSA is defined as repeated cessation of airflow in the lungs, and a concurrent cessation of respiratory effort. It usually affects older patients, and those who are undergoing CPAP for the first time as well as patients with high levels of CPAP pressure. CSA is also caused by high levels of Carbon Dioxide in the blood which results in hypercapnia. This is why we need to exhale CO_2 levels in our lungs, so that we can have normal levels of it in our blood. Occasional CSA is also common at the onset of sleep.

Central Sleep Apnea with Cheyne – Stokes Breathing

This is quite similar to what causes CSA but it is coupled with volume of breaths that forms a waning and waxing pattern which doctors see during the NREM or non – rapid eye movement. These waning and waxing patterns are usually corrected during the Rapid Eye Movement treatment. The common patients of Cheyne – Stokes breathing are senior male patients or those who are aged 60 and above. For a patient to be diagnosed as such, the pattern or the patient should have an average of 10 central apneas per hour of their sleep.

Central Sleep Apnea Caused by Medical Disorders without Cheyne – Stokes Breathing

Medical disorders like the so – called Degenerative Brainstem Lesions are known to contribute to central respiratory events wherein it becomes a secondary disorder.

Central Sleep Apnea Caused by High – Altitude Periodic Breathing

This occurs when the central apneas and hypopneas of patients are raised whenever they reached an altitude of around 4,000 meters (12,000 feet). This often occurs around 5 times per hour of sleep. Central events such as this tend to correct itself once the person is returned to lower altitudes, and it is also considered a normal adjustment.

Central Sleep Apnea Caused by Medication Intake

Drugs such as hydrocodone and methadone can sometimes cause central respiratory events, but in this case, the CSA is just secondary disorder.

Primary Central Sleep Apnea (in Infants)

Another life – threatening disorder characterized under CSA is called the Primary Central Sleep Apnea. This occurs when babies have long respiratory events that are central or obstructive in nature, and something that lasts for about 20 seconds or so. It can be very dangerous for newborn babies, and doctors should be able to diagnose it and treat the soonest.

Primary Central Sleep Apnea in Premature Infants

CSA is also quite common in babies who are born premature. If this is the case, the newborn infants will usually require ventilator support. For premature babies to be diagnosed with primary central sleep apnea, they should be less than 37 weeks old, and has a recurring central apnea of around 20 seconds for the duration of their sleep.

Treatment Emergent Central Sleep Apnea

This is also known as Complex Sleep Apnea, and it is usually diagnosed with OSA. The patient often times also had subsequent positive airway pressure or PAP. It occurs after solving obstructive events during the titration process, and it persists with around 5 central events per hour of sleep. Doctors treat patients using the bi - level PAP with a backup rate to resolve central events. Complex sleep apnea is now more prevalent among patients who are undergoing OSA treatments.

Sleep – Related Hypoventilation Disorders

Another type of sleep – related breathing disorder is known as sleep – related hypoventilation disorders. There are various classifications under this type which will be discuss in this section.

Obesity Hypoventilation Syndrome

This syndrome is also known as Hypercapnic Sleep Apnea, and formerly known as Pickwickian Syndrome although the latter term is not preferred because it used to describe patients who also have Obstructive Sleep Apnea. It is defined as hypoventilation that happens when the patients sleep.

Congenital Central Alveolar Hypoventilation Syndrome

This type of hypoventilation disorder is defined as the failure of the body's automatic central control of breathing, and it's usually due to a genetic mutation of a certain PHOX2B gene. Patients who have this kind of disorder usually experiences hypoventilation whenever they wake up (which is much worse than during their sleep) and at the onset of sleep.

Late – Onset Central Hypoventilation with Hypothalamic Dysfunction

Patients with this kind of disorders are usually healthy until around 2 years old or unless they become severely obese, then that's the time the onset of central hypoventilation takes place. The symptoms can be diagnosed during the first few years of the child, and it includes obesity, lack of gene mutation (PHOX2B), and other sleep – related hypoventilation disorders.

Idiopathic Central Alveolar Hypoventilation

This is also formerly referred to as alveolar hypoventilation or central alveolar hypoventilation. This type is characterized by the presence of alveolar ventilation that can result to sleep – related hypercapnia as well as hypoxemia in patients. Doctors diagnose this type of disorder by checking if there's a presence of sleep – related hypoventilation, but it's not due to other factors like medications or medical disorders.

Sleep – Related Hypoventilation Caused by Substance or Medications

This disorder is when the hypoventilation occur can be due to intake of medication or can be traced back from taking substances that can inhibit respiration, and is not something that is due to a medical disorder.

Sleep – Related Hypoventilation Caused by Medical Disorder

This disorder is when the hypoventilation that occurs can be traced back to a certain condition that can inhibit respiration, and is not something that is due to a substance or medicine intake.

Isolated Symptoms

Snoring

Snoring is when a person creates audible vibrations in their upper lungs whenever they inhale or exhale during their sleep. It is caused by partial obstruction in the lung's upper airway that may include nasal obstructions. Snoring can sometimes lead to having a dry mouth or throat irritation. In most cases, snoring can be so loud that it wakes up or disturb the other sleepers in the next room. It tends to increase if a person becomes slightly fat or when the person has obstructive sleep apneas since snoring is one of the common symptoms.

Snoring is usually corrected using CPAP, special sleep devices, dental appliances and devices that helps pull the lower jaw forward, and other snoring treatments like throat lubricants, pillar implants that's often inserted into the palate's soft tissues, and specialized pillows. The treatment and its effectiveness highly varies and depends on the condition of the patient as well as its characteristics.

Catathrenia

Also known as sleep – related groaning, and this happens when there's a repeated groaning when a person exhales during their sleep (occurs in Rapid Eye Movement). This is not entirely a disorder, and is more common in men than in women. Often the people beside the one groaning are disturb as a result.

Chapter Three: Central Disorders of Hypersomnolence & Circadian Rhythm Sleep – Wake Disorders

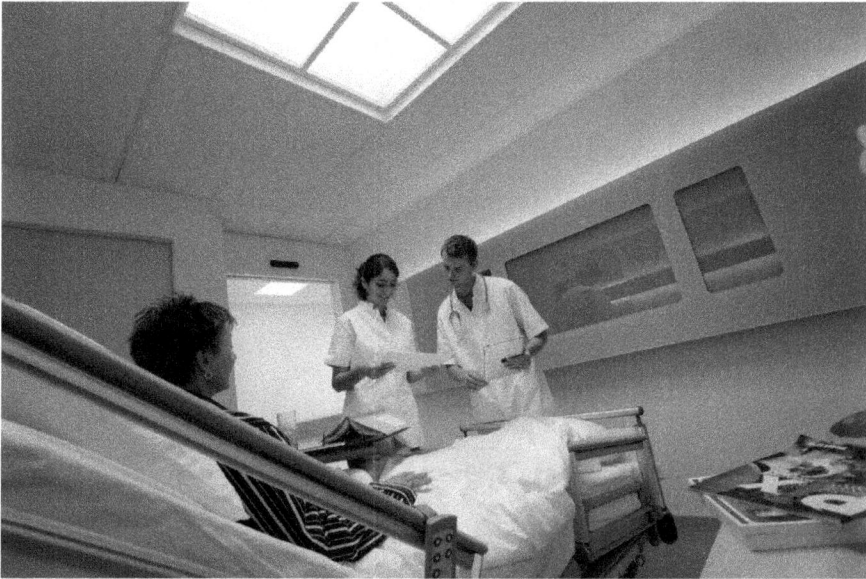

In this chapter, you'll learn other types of sleep disorders. The first one is categorized under the Central Disorders of Hypersomnolence; this is divided under many sub – types including Narcolepsy (Types I and II), Idiopathic Hypersomnia, and Kleine – Levin Syndrome as well as some of its causes. You'll also get to learn about the Circadian Rhythm Sleep – Wake Disorders which is also divided under different sub – types including the Delayed Sleep – Wake Phase Disorder, the Advanced Sleep – Wake Phase Disorder, Irregular Sleep – Wake Rhythm, the Non – 24 – hour – sleep – wake rhythm disorder just to name a few.

Central Disorders of Hypersomnolence

The sub – types that are included in this group of
sleep disorders are characterized as the primary complaint
in daytime sleepiness among patients which are not
necessarily due to misaligned circadian rhythms or
disturbance in night sleep. What medical practitioners use to
determine or diagnose which sub – type their patient
belongs to is through giving them the MWT (Maintenance of
Wakefulness Test, or the MSLT (Multiple Sleep Latency
Test).

Narcolepsy Type I

The first sub – category under the Central Disorders
of Hypersomnolence group is the Narcolepsy. It came from
the root words "narke and lepis" in Greek which means
numbness and attack respectively. As the root word
suggests, narcolepsy refers to the patient experiencing "sleep
attacks" and its main cause is either a pathological or
physiological abnormality. Symptoms include EDS
(excessive daytime sleepiness), Rapid Eye Movement sleep
phenomenon such as sleep paralysis and hypnogogic
hallucinations as well as cataplexy. Of course, the symptoms

varies from one patient to another depending on how severe or complicated there condition is.

The four common symptoms aforementioned created the so – called narcolepsy tetrad, and are major indicators that a patient has narcolepsy. Not a lot of patients experience all the symptoms at once although most suffer from more than one of the four mentioned earlier. Other common symptoms include irresistible napping or frequent napping, and what doctors call "automatic behavior." About 30 – 40% of narcoleptic patients experience automatic behavior; this is the subconscious performance of certain activities in an individual. These activities seemed like it is being done deliberately even when it's usually not or the patient has relatively no control over it. For instance, when the person speaks out of content on a particular subject matter and he/she didn't mean to do so, the individual may already exhibit narcolepsy.

Excessive Daytime Sleepiness

Let's go back to EDS or Excessive Daytime Sleepiness. It's another common symptom usually seen in most narcoleptic patients, and it manifests itself in various ways including but not limited to the following:

- Difficulty remaining awake during daytime
- Memory Loss

- Difficulty in concentrating which leads to poor performance
- Frequent napping in normal waking hours
- Reduced Cognition and performance in work – related tasks
- Hallucinations

EDS can also affect the patient's relationships, increase risk for automobile accidents (most narcoleptics fall asleep while driving), or work – related accidents. Patients are usually aware if there's an incoming "sleep attack" but they also can't help to unintentionally fall asleep at inappropriate times like in between conversations, while at work, or during sexual activity. Those who were able to fight off their sleep attacks may still experience episodes of the so – called "microsleep." As the name suggests, it is a very brief period of sleep that most patients experience. It is so short of a time that most patients aren't even aware that it happened. Some doctors say that this is a phenomenon where the individual feels a brief lack of awareness or consciousness. Doing short naps at some point during the day can help narcoleptics with EDS and microsleep symptoms.

Cataplexy

Another well – known symptom among narcoleptic patients is called cataplexy which came from the Greek words "Kata" and "Plexis."This means down, and seizure respectively. Most times, this phenomenon is mistaken for a seizure activity because patients exhibit bilateral loss of their muscle tones that may be provoked because of strong emotions. It manifests in the body through feeling of mild muscle weakness to complete limb atonia that often results from the person falling. Narcoleptic patients experiencing cataplexy symptom usually drops whatever they are holding which can oftentimes be embarrassing for them or harmful to others. Cataplexy symptom lasts for just a few seconds but can also be prolonged and caused periods of REM sleep.

About 70% of narcoleptic patients experience this symptom but they usually can fight it off through controlling their emotional stimuli.

Sleep Paralysis

This is defined as a partial to total paralysis of skeletal muscles once an individual wakes or at the onset of sleep. If it happens at the onset of sleep, the term is hypnagogic; on the other hand if it occurs upon waking up, the term is hypnopompic.

The sleep paralysis symptom is experienced by approximately 25% of narcoleptic patients that are usually linked with hypnagogic or hypnopompic hallucinations. It is often described as a dreamlike experience but it's very vivid, and with intense feeling of fear. Not everyone who experience sleep paralysis are considered narcoleptics because even normal people at some point have this kind of experience (though it could already be the start of the symptom's manifestation). It usually happens when a person is severely deprived of sleep. It is quite common in teenagers and those in their early 20's. At the time of this writing, there's still no known cure for sleep paralysis but treatments are now available to reduce or fight off this symptom of narcolepsy.

Causes of Narcolepsy

The exact cause of narcolepsy is not known but according to medical researchers, genes appear to be a strong component. Genetics play a role when it comes to the likelihood of a person developing narcolepsy. Based on research, narcoleptic patients also have increased amounts of dopamine, norepinephrine, and epinephrine in the brain. Sometimes head injuries and brain tumors can also cause a person to exhibit narcoleptic symptoms.

Most patients also suffer from depression due to the inability to carry out tasks at home or work, or do other normal activities. It can also cause them to have low self – confidence which is why most often than not, narcoleptics are underachievers.

Diagnosing Narcolepsy

Diagnosing an individual might be difficult because most of the symptoms can also be found in other relatively similar sleep disorders. Usually though, doctors will let the patient complete sleepiness tests, scales, or even let them do a sleep diary. They will also advise the patients to undergo an overnight diagnostic sleep study in order to rule out the symptoms of other sleep disorders like Obstructive Sleep Apnea. MSLT should also be carried out, it is a test that consists of a series of 5 short nap opportunities wherein the patient is given a time to fall asleep during these time periods. Rapid Eye Movement can occur during the sleep onsets which are a major indicator that a patient is exhibiting narcolepsy.

Sleep Onset REM periods or SOREMPs are also used to indicate a narcoleptic patients. Aside from all these, doctors will also diagnose the patient through their medical history, various physical exams, and sleep study questionnaires/ results.

Treating Narcolepsy

There are various behavioral and medical treatments that have been developed and have proven to be effective in helping the patients treat the symptoms. Such behavioral treatment for instance is taking short but regularly scheduled naps at some point during the day. Based on research it has been very effective in treating narcoleptic patients. Aside from this, it can also be helpful if the patient openly discuss or share their sleeping disorder to their family and friends or even colleagues so that they'll be aware of why they will sometimes do certain things or exhibit symptoms of the disorder. This can relieve the possibility of embarrassment or stress, and can help in preventing depression as well as underperformance.

Practicing proper sleep hygiene is another very beneficial and effective way to improve the quality of one's sleep (not just for narcoleptic/ sleep – disorder patients but also for normal sleepers) and also improve the ability to initiate and maintain sleep so that one can be awake and alert during the day.

Aside from these behavioral modifications, doctors also advise patients to use certain medications to treat and help ease the symptoms. The most common medicines for narcoleptic patients are CNS stimulants and Amphetamine - like medicines including Dexedrine, Provigil, Ritalin, Methamphetamine and Methylphenidate. CNS stimulants are usually prescribed to narcoleptic patients with EDS while suppressants and antidepressants are prescribed to those with symptoms of cataplexy, sleep paralysis, and hypnagogic hallucinations. Just recently, oxidase inhibitors and fluoxetine have been proven beneficial in also treating cataplexy.

Narcolepsy Type II

This is very similar to narcolepsy type I except for the fact that the cataplexy symptom is not present or being experienced by patients. Aside from the metrics mentioned above, it is often diagnosed through using a CSF or Cerebrospinal Fluid.

Idiopathic Hypersomnia

Another type under the Central Disorders of Hypersomnolence is called Idiopathic Hypersomnia. This is defined as the occurrence of refreshing naps, decreased sleep latency, and absence of cataplexy. The symptoms are usually secondary to other sleep disorders, and doctors diagnose it by checking if there's an absence of other symptoms from other sleep disorders.

Kleine – Levin Syndrome

This is also known as Periodic Hypersomnolence or Recurrent Hypersomnia. It happens when a patient experiences series of episodes of excessive sleeping or hypersomnia. Most patients classified under this category sleep most of the time (around 16 to 18 hours). They also exhibit symptoms of confusion and hallucinations. This kind of episode may last for 10 days to about a month and happens again at least once a year.

Causes of Hypersomnia

Hypersomnia Caused by Medical Disorders

It only happens when there's a primary medical condition that becomes the underlying cause for hypersomnia. The daytime sleepiness therefore is caused by a medical disorder.

Hypersomnia Caused by Substances or Medicine in - Take

Hypersomnia happens when there is substance or medication abuse that causes a person to have extended house of sleep or excessive sleep. It can also be a side – effect to some certain medications prescribed.

Hypersomnia with Psychiatric Disorder

Patients with psychiatric disorders usually meet the diagnostic criteria of hypersomnolence and can cause daytime sleepiness. It's quite prevalent with patients experiencing mood disorders including bipolar disorder, depression, and seasonal affective disorder.

Insufficient Sleep Syndrome

This is another common sleep disorder under this category that's also being experienced by normal people. It simply means that the individual is not sleeping long enough to satisfy one's physical and psychological needs. Other terms for this include Sleep Restriction or Chronic Sleep Deprivation. Some symptoms include daytime lapses, absence of other sleep disorders or medical disorders that could cause symptoms, and the likes. Common treatments include sleep pattern recording using the so – called actigraphy. This condition is very common in teenagers when the need for sufficient sleep is high but the lifestyle restricts it.

Circadian Rhythm Sleep – Wake Disorders

These are disorders wherein it is described as a disruption to one's normal circadian or body rhythm that causes individuals to experience symptoms like EDS, and insomnia or sometimes both. This is when your sleep schedule is not consistent where it can greatly disrupt your ability to fall asleep, maintain asleep that's required, and achieve a restorative kind of sleep that gets you going. There are several sub – types under this category of sleep disorder and that's what we're going to talk about in the next few sections.

Delayed Sleep – Wake Phase Disorder

This is described as a later sleep schedule than expected or desired by an individual. When a patient is diagnosed with this kind of circadian rhythm disorder, the person will be unable to fall asleep at their desired time or the normal bedtime, though they'll be able to sleep at a somewhat later time; this is why the patient usually wakes up late in the daytime. It's quite common in teenagers and young adults because they may have created a habit of staying up late at night. However, this is not something to worry about. Adopting proper sleeping hygiene can eventually lessen this kind of phase disorder.

Advanced Sleep – Wake Phase Disorder

This is quite the same with Delayed Sleep – Wake Phase Disorder but only this time a person falls asleep earlier that what one expects or desires. If a patient has this then he/she will have a hard time staying awake until his/her expected or normal bedtime and they tend to wake up too early in the morning. This is quite prevalent in older people who developed the habit of eating and sleeping early when they were younger. Again, this is not totally something to worry about and perhaps it's quite normal for teens and older people to experience these kinds of circadian rhythm disruption because of their chosen lifestyles. Adopting proper sleeping hygiene can definitely help if one needs to adjust their sleeping time.

Irregular Sleep – Wake Rhythm Disorder

It is described by having abnormal sleeping patterns and abnormal waking times. Although the total sleep time is almost the same with normal sleeping time, their sleep periods usually comes in forms of having plenty of naps as opposed to just remaining asleep for a certain period. Patients also exhibit episodes of insomnia and excessive daytime sleepiness or EDS.

Non – 24 Hour Sleep – Wake Rhythm Sleep Disorder

This is formerly referred to as "Free – Running Disorder." It is when the body's circadian rhythm is inconsistent with the 24 – hour clock. The circadian rhythm of patients experiencing this disorder is usually longer than 24 hours, and is not related to the light – dark cycle. Patients that are blind are usually the ones who experience this kind of circadian rhythm disorder.

Shift Work Disorder

As the name suggests, patients suffering from this disorder are those who are assigned in a so – called "graveyard shift" where they need to work during the wee hours of the morning, and very late at night. As a result of their work shift, their circadian rhythm are disrupted which is why they experience EDS. This kind of work requirement in the long run often results to poor work performance, reduced wakefulness, and impaired judgment. The people affected by this are those working in call centers, nurses in hospitals, and other on – call type of jobs. If a person wants to avoid this kind of disorder in the long – term then he/she needs to find a job where there's no night shift schedule assignment, or adapt a certain sleeping hygiene. Medical researchers carry out lots of studies about the negative effects of people who work in graveyard shifts.

Jet Lag Disorder

This happens when an individual travels in more than 2 time zones. It can result to insomnia, gastrointestinal disturbances, and EDS. It can also result to poor performance if one always travels across different countries all the time.

Circadian Rhythm Sleep Disorder Not Otherwise Specified

These kinds of disorders are characterized by a disruption of the body's normal circadian rhythm but don't meet the criteria of the aforementioned disorders. Usually it happens as secondary effects to certain medical disorders or due to medication in – take/ substance abuse. Some of this conditions that can produce disruption of the circadian rhythm are the following:

- Alzheimer's Disease
- Dementia
- Parkinson's Disease

Chapter Four: Parasomnias

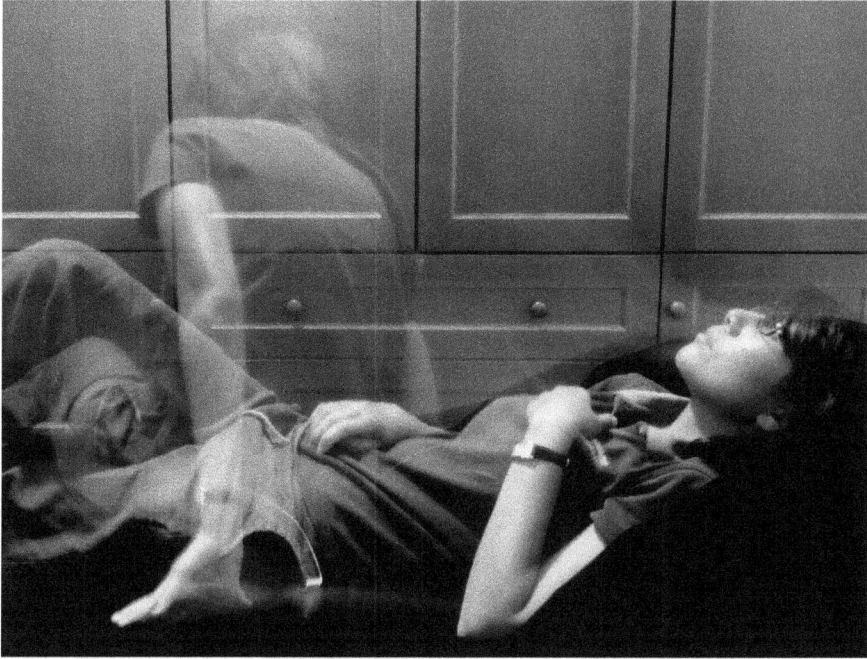

Parasomnia is one of the most commonly known sleeping disorders because some people relate this phenomenon to the 'unknown' or in relation to the spirits. This disorder is characterized by unwanted physical actions during sleep. A person is experiencing parasomnia whenever he/she is sleep walking, talking or has the so – called sleep terrors. According to science, this form of sleep disorder is associated with the rapid eye movement and the arousals from the non – rapid eye movement that can bring about such feelings or experiences, and is not something that's related to the spiritual realm.

This chapter will provide you with information regarding the different sub - types of parasomnias and also the different categories under each sub – types of disorders. The 2 categories under parasomnias are the Non Rapid Eye Movement – Related Parasomnias, and the REM or Rapid Eye Movement – Related Parasomnias. There are also other lesser known sub – types that you will later learn in this chapter.

Disorders of Arousal from Non – Rapid Eye Movement Sleep

The disorders under this sub – type includes Confusional Arousals, Sleep Walking, Sleep Terrors, and Sleep – Related Eating Disorder.

Confusional Arousals

This happens when an individual wakes up in a confused state. It usually occurs when the person wakes up from a slow wave sleep during the first third of the night, although it can still happen when one wakes up at any stage of their sleep. Once the person wakes up they tend to experience confusional arousal which means they might temporarily not know who they are, what's happening, or where they are. They may also tend to speak in a slurry way, and their mental process can become slow at the moment. If the person also suffers from hypersomnia or insomnia, then there could be an increase in experiencing confusional arousals. It may also be common among people who are deprived of sleep or those who have a shifting work.

Sleep Walking

Sleep walking occurs when certain behaviors such as sitting up, jumping, running, walking from bed happens during a slow wave sleep. Sleep walking can range from calm behaviors like just walking or sitting up to quite unusual and nasty behaviors like jumping off the house, running towards things and the likes. This is why sleep walking became quite popular since the behavior that's being exhibited is intriguing. Other very unusual behavior that occurs when a person is asleep which has been reported includes texting, sexual activities, and even committing murder. Sleep walking is quite common in children, and young adults or those in pre – pubescent stage.

Sleep Terrors

Also referred to as night terrors or nightmares; this is a disorder that happens when one is awaken from the slow wave sleep while experiencing feelings of intense fear. As you may know, such event usually starts with a cry or loud scream that can involve the person jumping out of bed or even doing violent actions. And when the person go back to sleep after waking up from their nightmares, they usually cannot remember what happened when they wake up in the morning.

Sleep – Related Eating Disorder

This is when the person has repeated instances of eating or drinking during arousals while they're still sleeping. This may often occur every night or at least many times per night. Usually patients experiencing this behavior eat junk foods or things that they don't typically eat/drink during the day. However, the danger is that if the patient lives alone, he/she can eat/drink harmful substances. Usually, patients eating/ drinking while sleeping are hard to wake up, and may not remember anything at all in the morning. As a result, some patients tend to gain weight due to high volumes of unhealthy food in – take at night.

Recurrent Isolated Sleep Paralysis

Sleep paralysis is usually a symptom of narcolepsy that happens when the person is unable to move during sleep (hypnagogic) or once they wake up (hypnopompic). This period usually lasts for a few seconds to a few minutes, and is quite common in narcoleptic patients. And because this is a symptom of narcolepsy but for a disorder called recurrent isolated sleep paralysis, it negates the diagnosis of a patient being narcoleptic. Unlike what most people believe, sleep paralysis is not caused by spirits or some kind of an element that tries to possess one's soul, it is simply due to shifting sleep habits, deprivation of sleep, and poor sleeping hygiene.

Nightmare Disorder

Just like sleep terrors, nightmares happen when a person had a bad dream that's usually very intense and scary which it causes one to become awake. And often times, when one does manage to wake up; they still feel the intensity of whatever they dreamed of. This occurrence is quite common in kids, and is also considered normal to them. When children reach a certain age, they may still experience nightmares every now and then but this time it's less intense and frightening. Normal adults may also from time to time experience this phenomenon and is also consider normal unless of course you are diagnose with having other mental disorders. It is a common symptom of PTSD or Post Traumatic Stress Disorder. Such patients experience nightmares that may result them to re – experiencing the frightening or intense events which can further worsen their condition as this event occurs during the Rapid Eye Movement Sleep phase where most dreaming usually takes place. Nightmares among PTSD patients give them a hard time falling back to sleep because they are still traumatized about their dreams.

Other Types of Parasomnias

Exploding Head Syndrome

This is a sleep disorder where a person experiences an imagined loud noise or a sense of explosion while they are asleep or upon awakening. Some patients also report that they see a flash of bright light while other report some sort of physical things as well. However, the person experiencing this may have no physical complaints or there are no malignant effects to their body but may have some form of pain in their head due to the loud noise they have upon awakening.

Sleep – Related Hallucinations

This is another common symptom found in narcolepsy. Both hypnagogic and hypnopompic hallucinations happen in narcoleptic patients wherein they experience a sort of visual hallucination when they wake up or when they fall asleep. Such hallucinations are usually linked with rapid eye movement periods that cause a person to become frightened and jump out of bed which can result to them injuring themselves. For doctors to diagnose a patient with sleep – related hallucinations, one should not have any other sleep disorders like narcolepsy because otherwise it will then be the diagnosis/ disorder. Sleep – related hallucinations often happen in young adults or teenagers, and it could also be a secondary issue for those suffering with dementia or Parkinson's disease.

Sleep Enuresis

This is also known as nocturnal enuresis. It happens when a person urinates several times while they sleep or the commonly known as bedwetting. Patients that usually experiences peeing in their beds do not respond to the sensations in the bladder that restricts the flow of urine and prevents them from wetting the bed. This is very common and normal in young kids, infants, and in elderly. For one to be diagnose with this disorder, they should be around 5 years old and below, and pees in the bed twice or more in a week. However, it can also happen to patients with post traumatic disorders, patients with diabetes, and those who are victims of abuse.

Causes of Parasomnias

Parasomnias Caused by Medical Disorder

Such disorder is only secondary because it is most likely due to a certain medical condition. Usually, parasomnia is experienced by patients diagnosed with dementia and Parkinson's disease that can also cause sleep – related hallucinations.

Parasomnias Caused by Medication in – take or Other Substances

Some parasomnias happen because of drug abuse or as a side – effect of certain medications like tricyclic antidepressants which are treatments for Alzheimer's disease. Huge consumption of caffeine can also cause parasomnia disorders.

Sleep Talking

Sleep talking is quite common and can happen in any age while a person is sleeping. It's also considered normal and benign because it can happen even to normal people who aren't diagnose with any sleep disorder or mental disorder. However, it may disturb other people in bed especially if the person is a loud sleep talker. Many people talk while sleeping without them being aware of it until their roommate informed them about it.

Chapter Five: Sleep – Related Movement Disorders

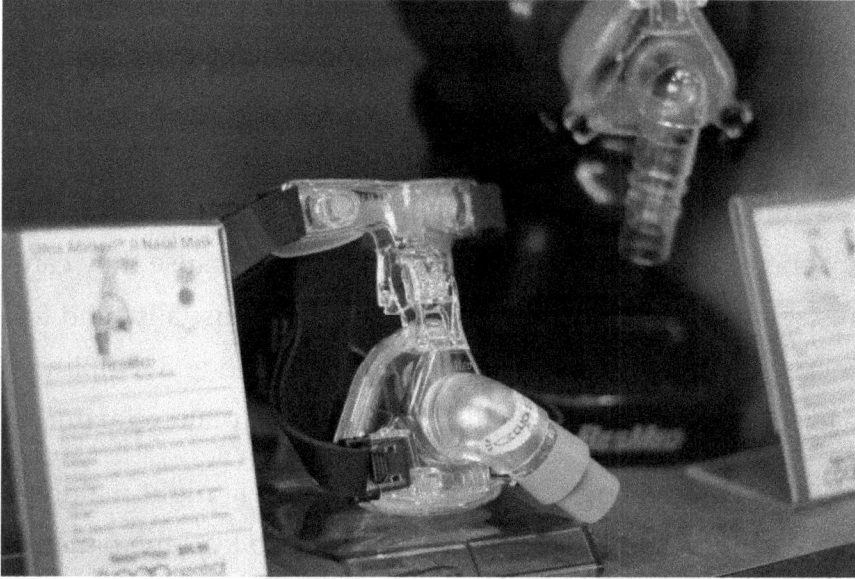

These kinds of disorders are usually described as something simple yet quite repetitive. Usually, people experiencing these kinds of disorder unconsciously move all the time when they are asleep causing their sleep to be disrupted, and also their bedmates to be disturbed. The sleep – related movement disorders include RLS or Restless Legs Syndrome, PLMD or Periodic Limb Movement Disorder, Sleep – Related Leg Cramps, Sleep – Related Bruxism, RMD or Rhythmic Movement Disorder, and BSMI or Benign Sleep Myoclonus of Infancy.

Restless Legs Syndrome

This is a kind of sleep – related movement disorder that's usually characterized by the body's urge to move in order to stop the odd sensations that usually can be felt in their legs. Such sensations (itchiness, crawling, tingling, creeping, burning feelings) can become really uncomfortable for them, which is why they need to move because they can't resist it. All of the feelings mentioned above usually tend to increase whenever the patient is in a relax mode like falling asleep, reading, sitting, watching TV or just plain relaxing.

These feelings are often experienced at night making them quite restless. This syndrome can also lead the patient to having insomnia.

Patients that are diagnosed with RLS will find themselves unable to resist twitching, slapping, jerking, and rubbing their leg muscles, bouncing in their feet, or even walk around just to alleviate the irresistible, restless, and uncomfortable feelings. Usually this kind of sensations lasts for a few seconds to even an hour!

RLS can happen at any age even in newborn babies. Usually though, RLS in children is misdiagnosed as growing pains or being hyperactive. Most patients start feeling these sensations of restlessness in their legs around their teenage years and progresses into adulthood. In the U.S. alone, 5% of the total population is diagnosed with restless legs syndrome. The frequency as well as the severity of this syndrome varies in patients depending if they have an underlying illness, pain or even if they are under stress. Sometimes pregnant women are also affected with this but it usually disappears after their pregnancy.

There are different diseases that may be linked with having RLS including OSA (obstructive sleep apnea), diabetes, rheumatoid arthritis, Parkinson's disease, iron deficiency, and other medical conditions. It may also result as a side – effect if the patient is taking certain medications like antidepressants, antipsychotics, and antihistamines.

Doctors usually prescribe dopamine, anticonvulsants, agonists, benzodiazepines, and opioids as treatment to RLS. They may also recommend other alternative treatments like massages, and musculoskeletal manipulations.

Most of the time, RLS patients aren't aware that they have this kind of disorder which is why it's very essential for sleep technicians to take note of such in order to address the issue. Most RLS patients also suffer from PLMD or Periodic Limb Movement Disorder which is what we will talk about next.

Periodic Limb Movement Disorder

Also known as Periodic Limb Movement in Sleep or PLMS, and formerly referred to as nocturnal myoclonus, is another common sleep disorder that is characterized when a patient involuntarily moves their legs or limbs while they are asleep. It is quite prevalent in senior patients or those who are 60 years old and above. In fact, 1/3 of them experience this along with other symptoms that are quite similar with RLS because the movements are also repetitive, but the difference is that it happens in periodic episodes. PLMD occurs mostly in stage N2 and not typically seen in Rapid Eye Movement sleep. Common symptoms include the following:

- Fragmented sleep
- EEG arousals
- Daytime sleepiness
- Stress and medications such as tricyclic antidepressants

PLMD affects not just the patient itself because their sleep is disrupted but also their bedmate because they can always be kicked at night.

The usual treatment given for PLMD patients includes medications like benzodiazepines and also dopaminergic. Such medications are able to suppress muscle contractions, and also regulate muscle movements while the patients are asleep. Anticonvulsants are also prescribed to inhibit muscle contractions as well as GABA agonists since it helps in relaxing the muscle contractions.

Sleep – Related Leg Cramps

This kind of disorder is described as something intense because the patients usually feel a sudden burst of leg cramps while they sleep. Muscle cramps for normal people are already painful, what more for these patients. It usually disrupts their sleep, and makes them wake – up. This is quite common in older people but can also happen among babies and young children.

Sleep – Related Bruxism

Bruxism is the act of grinding one's teeth or the habit of jaw clenching while sleeping. This type of sleep disorder is often times discovered by the patient's dentist because there's evidence of teeth grinding. Just like other sleep disorders, teeth grinding or bruxism can disrupt their own sleep and that of others. At the same time, the patient can experience some form of headache or jaw soreness upon wakening, and also cause the teeth's enamel to wear down. Sleep – related bruxism is usually seen in kids and young adults who kind of grow because of the disorder. Most patients experience doing this in their lifetime, and what many people do to prevent such act is by using a mouth guard as it can help in preventing further teeth damage.

Medical professionals who are sleep specialists conducted a study among patients doing sleep – related bruxism; they did this through the use of EEGs, EOGs or Electro – oculograms, snore channel as well as chin EMG. According to their findings, whenever a patients does grind its teeth or clenches their jaws during sleep, lots of face muscles tightens including the jaw muscles, neck muscles, and head muscle. This causes disruption in different channels. Heavy or loud snoring also has the same effect which is why sleep technicians are advised to take notes of the snore because some patients also exhibit bruxism along with it.

Sleep – Related Rhythmic Movement Disorder

This is also referred to as head banging or body rocking during sleep. It is described as a series of repetitive body movements while a person is sleeping or whenever the patient is experiencing some form of drowsiness. The patients are typically seen rocking their bodies back and forth, and also constantly moving their heads, hence the name. This type of sleeping disorder is quite prevalent in newborns and weeks old infants but it is considered normal for them to do such rhythmic motions. Once they reach the age of 5 or older, the symptoms usually go away. As a result, such movements at night or during bedtime can cause disruption in one's sleep or harm the one sleeping beside them.

Benign Sleep Myoclonus of Infancy

Benign Sleep Myoclonus of Infancy or BSMI is also known as limb jerks; it is simply the various body movements while an infant is sleeping. However, it can affect any age, though it's quite prevalent in infants. The babies usually do repetitive leg jerks, but once they grow up, such movements do not occur. It also doesn't pose any serious threat to the baby's sleeping health though it could cause some occasional arousals.

Propriospinal Myoclonus at Sleep Onset

Propriospinal Myoclonus at Sleep Onset or PSM happens when there are repetitive body movements in the neck, abdomen, and also the trunk part of the person's body during sleep. It usually happens at sleep onset, and also during the short arousals from sleep.

Causes of Sleep – Related Movement Disorder

Sleep – Related Movement Disorder Caused by a Medical Disorder

This is when a sleep – related movement disorder is caused by a certain medical illness. It can be seen in conditions like the Parkinson's disease where there's an involuntary muscle movements that happens when the patient is sleeping, causing their sleep to be disrupted.

Sleep – Related Movement Disorder Caused by a Medication in – Take or Substance

This is when a sleep – related movement disorder is caused by use of certain medications and comes off as a side – effect. Sometimes it can be caused by substance abuse as well.

Isolated Symptoms of Sleep – Related Movement Disorder

The following group of sleep – related movement disorder has been classified as borderline abnormal but is not classified into specific disorders.

Excessive Fragmentary Myoclonus

This happens when the person is having frequent muscle twitches particularly in its fingers, mouth muscles, and toes upon awakening or while sleeping. Such movements though are benign, and is identifies as insignificant but can still be a symptom of other types of sleep disorder. The twitches happen during the Non – Rapid Eye Movement sleep, and lasts for about 20 minutes or so.

Hypnagogic Foot Tremor (HFT) and Alternating Muscle Activation (ALMA)

The hypnagogic foot tremor is when the legs or foot movements have a rhythmic pattern once they fall asleep or during sleep. On the other hand, alternating leg muscle activation is relative similar with HFT but the only difference is that one leg usually follows the movement of the other leg. Such movements can cause brief arousals, and sleep disruption but it's also benign in most patients experiencing it.

Hypnic Jerks or Sleep Starts

Hypnic jerks is characterizes as a sudden muscle movement or jerk at the onset of sleep, and it's usually accompanies by feelings of falling, fear, or surprise. It's benign for most patients but it can cause sleep disruption and difficulty to go back to sleep.

Other Type of Sleeping Disorders

There are certain sleep disorders that had just been discovered by medical researchers but is not yet classified under any sleeping categories because they overlap such categories or it's totally a new disorder. One of which is called the Environmental Sleep Disorder.

Environmental Sleep Disorder

According to sleep experts, environmental sleep disorder can consists of various factors such as making the bed partner hold the patient while sleeping which can cause sleep disruption. For instance, a PLMD patient's bedmate is also likely to experience some form of insomnia, EDS and even fatigue because of the sleep disruption due to the symptoms or body movements being exhibited by the PLMD patient. Other factors of environmental sleep disorder which can cause sleep disruptions include loud music, the room temperature, lighting, and even when one leaves their television on/off before going to bed.

Chapter Six: Alternative Medicine and Herbal Remedies

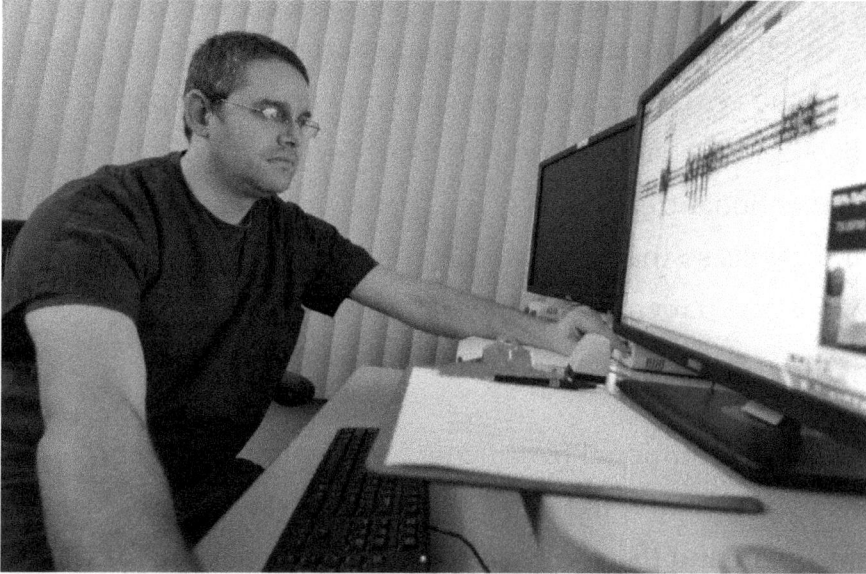

A normal sleep usually consists of 4 to 6 cycles that are categorized into two – the Non – Rapid Eye Movement (NREM) sleep and Rapid Eye Movement (REM sleep) as identified through the EEG or Electroencephalograph. According to medical researcher named Rechtschaffen, sleep is technically defined as the stage where there's a predominant pattern of epochs (eye movement, EEG, and muscle) for usually a period of 30 seconds. This chapter will focus on the different alternative treatments that one can do to help the symptoms of various sleeping disorders. It will also include information with regards to using herbal remedies as conducted by the Sleep Health Foundation.

Conventional Treatments vs. Unconventional Treatments

Before we discussed other alternative ways on how to treat the symptoms or occurrences of various sleeping disorders partially or completely, let's first discuss the conventional treatments given to patients and also its limitations so that you can fully understand the context of why some patients seek alternative remedies.

Conventional treatments for sleeping disorder like insomnia are divided into 2 types: the psychological treatment and the pharmacological treatment or medication in – take.

Psychological Treatment

Behavioral interventions or more commonly known as psychological treatments, aims to change the beliefs and habits of a patient diagnosed with insomnia or assumed to have other sleeping disorders. It typically includes three things namely; sleep restriction, stimulus control therapy, and sleep hygiene education. Many sleep specialists advocate doing a multi – dimensional treatment approach but unfortunately using pharmacological treatments like hypnotic agents prevail.

Pharmacological Treatment

Benzodiazepines

These are the most commonly prescribed drug for those patients diagnosed particularly with insomnia because it has constantly proven to be effective in treating the disorder for short – term. One of the side – effects of it however is that patients can experience a so – called anterograde amnesia and residual daytime drowsiness especially if it is a long – acting medication.

Tricyclic Antidepressants

These kinds of antidepressants are also what most doctors prescribed for insomnia patients, and usually in doses because it's also used to treat depression. Unfortunately, there are only a few scientific researches that prove the safety and effectiveness of these drugs, and it often has some side – effects such as dry mouth, constipation, and urinary retention or other anticholinergic effects. It also causes sexual dysfunction, cardiac toxicity, and orthostatic hypotension.

Antihistamines

Most over – the – counter drugs contains an active agent called antihistamine. Its job is to antagonize the central receptors of the brain or the histamine. Most antihistamine drugs may actually reduce sleep quality and has minimal effect when inducing sleep among patients. It's generally safe to take but can still have anticholinergic side – effects like the things we've mentioned earlier.

Limitation in Drug Therapies

For those diagnosed with insomnia, doctors traditionally recommend the use of hypnotic drugs as treatment which usually is taken by the patient for 4 weeks or a month. This is because if it's taken for a longer period of time, there's a huge chance of the patient experiencing problematic withdrawal symptoms, and also habituation (they might become addicted to it). There are only a few studies conducted with regards to the safety and efficacy of using hypnotic drugs for more than 2 to 3 months but some insomnia patients (about 15%) have already tried using the medication for about a year, so it the possible side – effects is perhaps a case to case basis. The most important thing is to consult your doctor first and follow their recommended time frame of hypnotic medication in – take.

Some doctors prescribed hypnotic drugs for the long – term as it can really help patients that are experiencing insomnia because of psychogeriatric factors. However, there are lots of patients who are experiencing side – effects and complications with regards to treating insomnia if hypnotic drugs are prescribed in the long run. Nevertheless, there are still constant studies about the ideal types of hypnotic drugs that can help patients maintain sleep, rapidly induce sleep, and also not have a hangover in the morning or upon wakening.

Alternative Therapies

Over – the – counter non – prescriptive medications have now become quite popular in relieving insomnia symptoms or helping one to fall and maintain quality sleep. According to a survey, about 10% of young adults used these non – prescriptive medications to improve their sleep. There have been quite a lot of patients who self – medicate using herbal remedies, amino acids, and also hormones so that they can have a quality sleep without experiencing the side – effects of sleeping pills or other prescribed medications. Usually, patients uses botanical based sleeping medicines such as Valerian, Hops, Passionflower and Kave to treat the sleeping disorder they may have particularly those with insomnia. Some patients also use various physiological substances to aid in their sleeping such as melatonin and hydroxytryptophan while other try Chinese Medicine therapies like acupuncture, and also the so – called low energy emission therapy.

Herbal Remedies for Sleep Disorders

There are essential things you need to know about using herbal medicines when it comes to alleviating the occurrences of various symptoms of sleeping disorders. Take note of the following:

- Many patients prefer using herbal medicines when treating sleeping problems rather than synthetic sleeping pills since most herbal medicines have less side – effects, if not at all. However, your physician may prescribe you certain medications aside from getting therapies or treatments that could affect your condition if you drink or take herbal medicines. Therefore, it is always wise to consult first with your doctor, and talk to them the kinds of herbal medicines you're planning to take to avoid certain side – effects or overlapping with your current medication/therapy.

- There had been many research conducted about the benefits of various medicinal herbs but some of the studies may not have been carried out properly. Some herbs actually have no strong evidence that's backed by scientific data as to whether or not they are effective or beneficial to patients with certain sleeping disorders or symptoms. Again, it's best to consult your doctor and ask them what could also be the benefits or side – effects.

- Herbal medicines that were somewhat proven to be quite beneficial in relieving sleeping disorder symptoms and helping patients sleep better or have a quality sleep so far include herbs like Valerian, Kava, Hops, and Passionflower. However, there's also relatively an evidence of why these herbs are effective, and further studies needs to be done. Take it at your own risk and consult your doctor.

- There are certain risks involved when taking alternative medicines like herbs. It may be beneficial for some people, but may also not work for some. It will perhaps highly depend on the severity of one's sleeping disorder, or it's a case to case basis. It's best that you manage the risk with the help of your doctor if this is what you really prefer, and let go of it if you found out that it's not working for you after at some point in time.

Medicinal Herbs as Remedies

In this section, we'll take a closer look at some of the most common herbs used in treating insomnia and possibly other types of sleeping disorders.

Valerian (*Valeriana officinalis*)

In the United States, Valerian herbs were one of the best – sellers out of the 25 herbal medicines around 1996. *V. officinalis* which is the scientific name contains roots and rhizome that was initially used to aid in inducing sleep and as an anxiolytic. In fact, the use of Valerian herb dates back to about 1,000 years.

The reason why many patients use Valerian as an alternative is because it is rated GRAS or Generally Recognized as Safe by the Food and Drug Administration (FDA) in the U.S. It is also listed in the European Pharmacopeia, and is among the widely use daytime sedative and as a hypnotic.

Valerian contains things like valerenic acid, and valepotriates as well as other unidentified aqueous content that contributes to its sedative properties.

This medicinal herb has been shown to help induce sleep among patients, and it also has an anxiolytic and tranquilizing effects when it was tested clinically, and used in animal studies. It is placebo – controlled because there had been a study where about 400 mg of valerian extract was tried by about 130 volunteers and as a result it improved the quality of their sleep, reduced frequent night awakening, and also decreased sleep latency. Further, there are other clinical studies showing that valerian herb in – take improve insomnia. And when it is taken 3 times in a day (135 mg of aqueous dried extract of valerian herb), it can decrease Stage 1 sleep, and also improve delta sleep.

According to other clinical studies, the extracts of Valerian herb causes muscle relaxation and also CNS depression. Its sedating qualities inhibits enzyme – induced breakdown of GABA in a person's brain, which can cause sedation but there's quite an uncertainty about the availability of its sedation properties.

Valerian is generally safe and approved by the FDA but there have been reports here and there when it comes to its effectiveness and quality. Patients who are taking large doses of valerian extracts have been reported to experience a serious form of withdrawal symptoms especially if it's followed by a sudden discontinuation of use.

Overall, the valerian extract shows that it can help improve the quality of sleep, decrease sleep latency, and alleviate the experience of insomnia among patients with perhaps only mild hypnotic side – effects.

Ginseng

For around 2,000 years now, ginseng root is still one of the most used herbal because it contains various health – promoting properties. It's also constantly the top 10 best – selling herbs in the U.S. According to various clinical researches, ginseng can also contribute in maintaining quality and restorative sleep and wakefulness. There are many species of ginseng herb but the most effective when it comes to sleep modulation are the Panax Ginseng form Korea or Asia, Panax Quinquefolius from America, and Panax Vietnamensis from Vietnam. Ginseng contains the following components:

- Ginsenosides
- Polyacetylenic Alcohols
- Peptides
- Fatty Acids

In recent studies, ginseng can also influence the quality of life in urban dwellers. According to the study a daily in – take of 40 mg ginseng for around 3 months can significantly improve the quality of life including their sleep.

There are however, a few reports of the side – effects of ginseng extracts that's quite severe but still, around 6 million Americans take it regularly despite of the potential side – effects. Usually, it will cause a person to become nervous or very exhilarated but it goes away if the dose or frequency of in – take is reduced. When it comes to taking ginseng extracts for long – term usage, reports have concluded that ginseng doesn't have any serious adverse reactions making it generally safe.

Usually, the recommended daily dose is 1 to 2 grams of crude root or around 200 to 600 mg of ginseng extracts. Many authors also suggest limiting the intake to just about 12 weeks. It's best to consult your doctor before taking it.

Kava Kava (Piper methysticum)

Kava kava is a large shrub that is usually found in the Pacific islands. When it comes to its therapeutic use, the rhizome of Kava kava is helpful in treating stress, anxiety disorders, and restlessness which is usually insomnia's underlying causes.

Kava kava contains kava lactones and kava pyrones which is a group of resinous compounds. Kava kava is also attributed with having central muscular relaxant effects, anti – convultion, antispasmodic, and acts as a sedative as well. In animal trials, it also shows that the extracts of it induces sleep and muscle relaxation. According to researchers, the underlying mechanism of this herb is not entirely clear and still needs further studies but it's possible that the extracts bind sites in the brain's GABA. There had been short – term clinical research providing that Kava kava is quite effective in relieving insomnia and anxiety, though the evidence is still relatively low and need further research.

As a sleeping aid, most patients take around 180 to 210 mg of kava lactones every day. Consult your doctor.

Passion flower (Passiflora incarnata)

The herb consists of a fruiting tip of the perennial climbing vine and also dried flower. The only downside is that this herb lacks enough evidence and studies to prove its efficacy but despite of that some people still find it useful in treating insomnia. The active components of this herb include harmala – type indolealkaloids, ethyl – maltol, maltol, and also flavonoids. When it was tried in animal teting, passion flower extract has significantly prolonged effects to the sleeping time of the rats tested. Patients take 4 to 8 grams of passion flower and it's usually taken as a tea. However, its harmala compounds are uterine stimulants, which is why it's not recommended for pregnant women. Side – effects have not been reported and also needs further research.

Hops (Humulus lupulus)

Another popular sleep herb is the dried strobili of Hops. It's been used for many centuries but as an intestinal illnesses treatment. Recently though, it's been used as a sedative – hypnotic. The component that's found in this herb includes estrogenic substances, flavonoids, volatile oil, tannins, and valerianic aci. Its sedative effects have been demonstrated to induce quality sleep.

For those patients with insomnia, they usually take it as a tea, and are quite effective in helping digestion around 20 to 40 minutes of intake. The recommended daily dose (sometimes several times a day) is 0.5 grams. There had been no proven side – effects but it's not recommended for pregnant women because it has estrogenic substances that can bring about estrogen – dependent breast cancer.

Physiological Alternative Treatments

Melatonin

This is a hormone in the body that's secreted in the pineal gland of the brain, and it's considered as a natural body remedy for those experiencing insomnia due to circadian schedule changes like shifting work or jet lag. Rapid time zones across different countries can result in the de – synchronization of the intrinsic human circadian or body rhythm as well as the environmental photoperiod. The severity and duration of the sleep disturbances vary depending on how many time zones a person crossed, the departure time, age, and also direction of travel. One study found out that after a 9 day round trip from New Zealand to Los Angeles to Great Britain, 2 of the flight – crew members being studied had less jet lags after taking melatonin.

Melatonin according to Folkard et al., said that the in – take of melatonin increases the quality of sleep when it was a test is carried out with night – shift workers as the subject. It also has shown many beneficial effects to older patients diagnosed with insomnia. However, there had been some adverse effects such as depression, headaches, tachycardia, pruritus, and sedation in the clinical trials.

The optimal dosing is quite unclear and the mechanism of its effectiveness is not yet known. Melatonin may be effective for patients with insomnia but further research is needed particularly when it comes to the toxicity and its efficacy.

L – Tryptophan and 5 – Hydroxytryptophan

L – tryptophan is an amino acid that's mostly found in plants and some animals. A dose of 1 g of it has been reported to reduce sleep latency and also reduce waking time. The amino acids acts like a serotonin which can improve the function of brain cells causing it to induce sleep among patients. However, you need to get a doctor's prescription before you can buy and take this physiological treatment as it was previously recalled by the FDA back in 1989 due to an incident.

On the other hand, 5 – Hydroxytryptophan is also currently used as a to treat depression, lose weight, and also as a sleeping aid. Taking in 100 mg of it daily increases slow

– wave sleep but it's not yet confirmed by controlled therapeutic studies. Make sure to consult your doctor first.

Other Alternative Approach

Acupuncture

Acupuncture is a form of therapy in Traditional Chinese Medicine. It has also become quite popular in the U.S. as an alternative therapy for all sorts of diseases and disorders. Moreover, the main use of acupuncture in Chinese Medicine is actually to treat insomnia.

According to clinical research in United States, acupuncture therapy has proven its efficacy in treating insomnia among psychiatric patients. There had been various controlled medical tests that demonstrate its effect. In fact, a recent study has shown that those patients with primary insomnia have improved both objectively and subjectively when it comes to the quality of their sleep.

Positive effects were shown almost after the treatment itself. Acupuncture usually involves the placing of needles in various points of the body, and for treating insomnia; the points will be in the scalp, ears and other body parts.

Low Energy Emission Therapy (LEET)

Low Energy Emission Therapy is a method that delivers low levels of amplitude – modulated radio frequency electromagnetic fields to patients. The device use for this procedure typically consists of a microprocessor, amplifier and signal generator. The signal generator is a connected to a mouthpiece that's held between the patient's palate and tongue for the treatment's duration. Recent studies suggest that LEET procedure can actually be an alternative therapy for those with chronic insomnia. Among the healthy volunteers they have tested, in just about 15 minutes of LEET procedure, there had been a changed in the EEG that's objectively and subjectively linked with relaxed feelings.

The mechanisms of LEET treatment are not yet fully understood. This is why the administration of this procedure is only limited to sleep disorder centers. Compared to conventional therapies, LEET can be done on an every other day basis. Moreover, there had been known induce bound insomnia if the treatment is discontinued. There also has no reported or proven side – effects of LEET as of this writing.

FAQs in taking Herbal Medicines to Treat Sleeping Disorders

Why should I try herbs? Can it really make me sleep better?

It's entirely up to you if you want to consider taking an alternative treatment like herbal medicines. In fact, about 40% of patients would like to try if herbal medicines will work for them, including those diagnosed with sleeping disorders, and also those people who just wanted to have a quality and restorative sleep because it is a complementary medicine, and may have less to no side effects in the long run compared to taking sleeping pills or other similar types of medications.

Are herbs really effective in helping treat sleeping disorders? Are there any related studies being done to prove its effectiveness?

As previously mentioned, there had been countless studies about certain herbs that could help in treating sleeping disorders and other illnesses. However, such studies and research may not always be complete and thorough. For some people it may work just fine but it's also important to notice if such effects aren't only a placebo/ dummy effect because the patient believe that it will heal them, similar to when patients took sugar pills and researchers made them believe that it's a beneficial medicine/ herb. There had been many studies about herbal remedies that failed the test of the placebo treatment. Unfortunately, there aren't any solid evidence or proof about the effectiveness of herbal medicines and this is mostly because such herbs can't be patented, trial testing are usually expensive, and not having a claim or patent over the data they've gathered means that research companies will conduct it at the expense of their investment even if certain herbs have potential. You may still encounter different clinical research and trials but again it may not be thorough. Some clinical studies have shown that herbs like the things we've mentioned earliest can help patients diagnosed with anxiety and insomnia.

What is any of the existing evidence say about certain herbs with regards to it helping patients sleep better?

The table below will show you the effectiveness of the 9 herbs in helping treat insomnia. We'd like to point out that the data given here is based from the research conducted by the Sleep Health Foundation, and the author and publisher of this book have no claim over this research. This is only used as a reference to inform and educate the readers of the possible benefits of the herbs listed below for those patients diagnosed with insomnia:

Herbal Medicine	Supported by clinical trials?	Supported via animal/ test tube studies?	Evidence level or effectiveness level for treating insomnia?
Kava (Piper Methysticum)	Yes	Yes	Needs further research
Valerian (Valerian spp.)	Yes	Yes	Low
Passionflower (Passiflora spp.)	Yes	No	Low
Hops (Humulus Lupulus)	Yes	Yes	Needs further research
Sour Date (Zizyphus	No	Yes	Needs further

Jujube)			research
Mimosa (Albizia Julibrissin)	No	Yes	Low
Lavender (Lavendula spp.)	No	Yes	Needs further research
California Poppy (Eschscholzia Californica	No	Yes	Needs further research
Chamomile (Matricaria Recutita)	No	No	Needs further research

As you can see in the table above, it is arranged in order of the strength of the evidence that they are effective (from strongest to the least). The first column shows if the herb is found to work well when it was tested with humans, and it also compares the herb to a placebo effect. This is perhaps the best type of study because it will really show whether it is beneficial or not. The second column shows the laboratory findings when the herbs were tested in animals or through test tube based examinations. However, the evidences based on this research conducted are not as relatively strong compared to a human type of trial. The third column shows the strength of the results as conducted across all the tests done for insomnia. There are 3 possible levels of evidence that can be found. The level of effectiveness is determined; if such studies and trials done has consistently good results. If the results are mixed but mostly well, the level will be Medium, but if there's a mix of both equally good and bad results, then the level will be Low.

As you refer back to the table listed, the first four of the nine herbs have shown beneficial to helping treat insomnia based on the human clinical trials. These are Passionflower, Hops, Kava and Valerian. Three of the four herbs also have good results when it was tested to animals and laboratory studies. The third column summarizes the evidence of the test results and also the level of the supporting evidences when it comes to treating insomnia. As you can see, it is Low and almost all herbs need further research. The research among these herbs in general haven't yet reached a conclusion as to what the actual benefits are or the roles of each in treating insomnia or perhaps other sleeping disorder. It is insufficient and the research also lacks quality making the effectiveness of these herbs to treating insomnia fairly weak.

Can herbs also help treat anxiety disorders?

It is a fact that some people are having a hard time falling asleep, maintaining asleep, and even having a restorative sleep because of anxiety. Clinical trials have once again relatively shown that there are a few herbs that may very well reduce anxiety, and in turn can help patients sleep better. Such herbs include Passionflower, Chamomile, and Kava. In fact, it was concluded that Kava had a relatively high evidence of effectiveness when it comes to reducing anxiety effects. On the other hand, Chamomile and Passionflower have Medium evidence levels.

What are the factors that can affect the results of the research?

Not all researchers and studies obviously have the same methods when it comes to selecting certain factors for their study, and some might not even thoroughly assess all the types of insomnia. It is possible though that herbal medicines or remedies may be more effective for some types of insomnia but it will need further research. Some studies may also not use the same amount of herb extracts.

Do herbal medicines or herbal remedies work right away?

There had been studies where the effects of such herbs take a few weeks before seeing any significant changes. Of course, it's best to not expect that you'll see any changes overnight or even just a few days after taking it. According to clinical research, the Valerian herb in particular, takes time before seeing its benefits kick in. Based on the trials conducted, it may take about a week or two before seeing any improvement in the patient's condition.

Are these herbal medicines safe to use?

Based on former clinical studies particularly a study review of the safety of Kava herb back in 2002, the herb's extract is safe for most users. However, this is only when taken in a period of time and at doses that are just enough. Some patients, unfortunately, found Kava to have side – effects in their bodies but further research needs to confirm this, because there are perhaps certain factors that aren't ruled out or the patient may have other underlying condition. Some studies also found out that Kave herb shouldn't be taken together with Benzodiazepines – which is a drug typically prescribed among patients diagnosed with sleeping disorders.

Conclusion

Conventional treatments for insomnia and sleep disorders usually involve taking various medications that may cause a depressant effect on the psychological therapy and the brain's CNS. It typically involves some risk such as addiction, or habituation, overdose, various side – effects, and drug tolerance. This is why alternative treatments such as herbal remedies, and other physiological agents are increasingly becoming popular because aside from the fact that they relieve symptoms and occurrences, most of them have less drawbacks as compared to using conventional drugs. However, the efficacy of these alternative treatments will still need further research to be fully understood.

Chapter Seven: The Future of Sleep Disorder Treatments

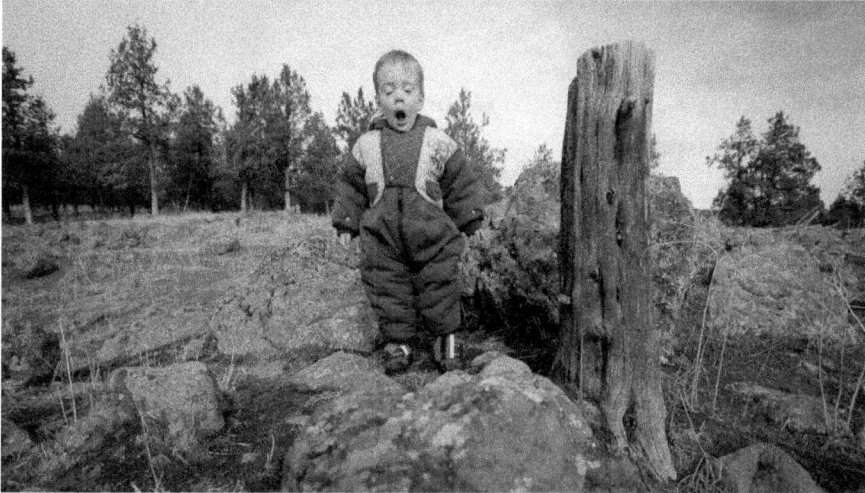

According to Dr. Charlene Gamaldo, medical director of John Hopkins Center for Sleep at the Howard County General Hospital, he said that the future of sleep research will look very different in the future as "Sleep clinical care and research is in a revolutionary place because of technology." You see most people knows what goes on during a sleep study test because doctors usually run night sleeping tests in the laboratory where patients or subjects are all wired up but because of the advent of technology as what Dr. Gamaldo said, there's a very high probability that the brick - and -mortar model of conducting sleep research in medical centers will eventually fade in the next few years as technology continues to become more and more advance. New studies will likely be conducted at the comfort of home.

The Future of Conducting Sleep Disorder Treatments

At – Home Sleep Testing Devices

Due to advances in technology, the sleep tests in the future will most likely be conducted at home using various high – tech sleep testing devices. It will be more common and could also be conventional. According to Dr. Gamaldo, there are now many portable devices being develop that are in line with the results or procedure being done in the laboratory that shows a lot of promise. Such technology and device can perhaps monitor the breathing of the patient while they are sleeping, and what's going on when a person is asleep without any wires attached to them. The FDA has approved many potential home devices to help monitor or diagnose sleeping disorders, and such devices can now measure the following:

- **Measure sleeps brain wave activity.** Most devices being develop today show doctors how a patient can quickly fall asleep, how deep they can sleep, and whether or not the sleep is restorative or if it's a quality kind of sleep.

- **Assess leg movements.** Some devices can now also detect quickly if a patient potentially has a restless leg syndrome or RLS.

- **Monitors breathing during sleep state.** Many devices being develop aims to help doctors diagnose patients with possible sleep apnea conditions.

Such portable monitoring at – home devices is very beneficial for doctors because it can capture the patient's natural sleeping pattern and what it's like when a person is in his/her own sleep environment compared to when the test is conducted in the laboratory where the patient is aware of what's happening. Plus it gives patients the ability of carrying out the various sleeping tests needed at the comfort of their own home or anywhere they want. While such portable at – home sleeping devices are becoming more and more accurate, people will still need to go to the laboratory if a more comprehensive test needs to be done. Sometimes there's also an advantage of carrying out such diagnostic exams in a controlled environment with a professional sleep technician and with a sleep specialist so that if something goes wrong someone can help a patient achieve more accurate results.

Phone Apps and Wearable Technology

Today's world is ruled by apps or applications that run on smartphones. Most people now use these apps in getting practically everything not just information but also things that helps us in our everyday lives. In medicine, particularly in the sleep research field, apps are also now being developed to help doctors and patients monitor sleep or detect any sleeping disorder. You can now use apps to record a person's snore which is usually a symptom of sleep apnea and is very common. Such feature can indicate the presence of certain sleep conditions that were once only conducted in sleep laboratories.

There are also various tracking devices or wearable technology in addition to apps that can help researchers and doctors alike in gathering information about their patients or subject's condition that were also once just gathered in a laboratory setting or controlled environment. Such devices are very convenient and can significantly increase the people's access to care, but app developers and gadget researchers will still need to ensure that the apps or devices they make have undergone various testing and there should be evidences that it works and it's accurate to prove that it can ultimately help people and sleep specialists in the future.

Telehealth

Telehealth is a type of communication technology that is now being developed further in order to reach more possible patients. It typically involves a video web conference where doctors and sleep specialists can help patients through online consultations with regards to their sleep health. It also provides researchers and clinicians to share data to one another to further their research. Telehealth will definitely become conventional in the future with the help of the internet and technology. This can help doctors reach patients living in far – off places who may not have a lot of medical options or health resources available in their area. It will help them connect to their doctors and treat their conditions in an easy, affordable and comfortable way.

Further Research about Sleeping Disorders

According to Dr. Gamaldo, sleep disorders are often times underdiagnosed, which is why researchers will need to find better ways in treating conditions especially the most common types such as insomnia, RLS or restless legs syndrome, and sleep apnea. Researchers will need to further study the effects of not getting enough sleep because chronic sleep deprivation or sleep loss is becoming an epidemic especially in the U.S.

According to statistics, more and more Americans are losing sleep every night making sleep disorders prevalent and severe more than ever. Sometimes it's unintentional because it is the kind of world we now live in; more people are now doing night shifts at work, some are binge watching online, spending lots of time in social medias, watching too much TV, or they are simply distracted by their phones and computers that it comes to a point where people are not getting adequate sleep every night due to these activities.

According to sleep doctors, the better and brighter screen that high – tech devices bring can cause damage to one's health, interfere with the body clock, and also promote bad sleeping hygiene or create sleeping disorders in the long run. Therefore, the challenge to researchers is to further study how the lack of sleep or poor quality sleep can impact a person's overall condition, affect their performance, and also bring about other illnesses like heart diseases and diabetes.

Chapter Summary

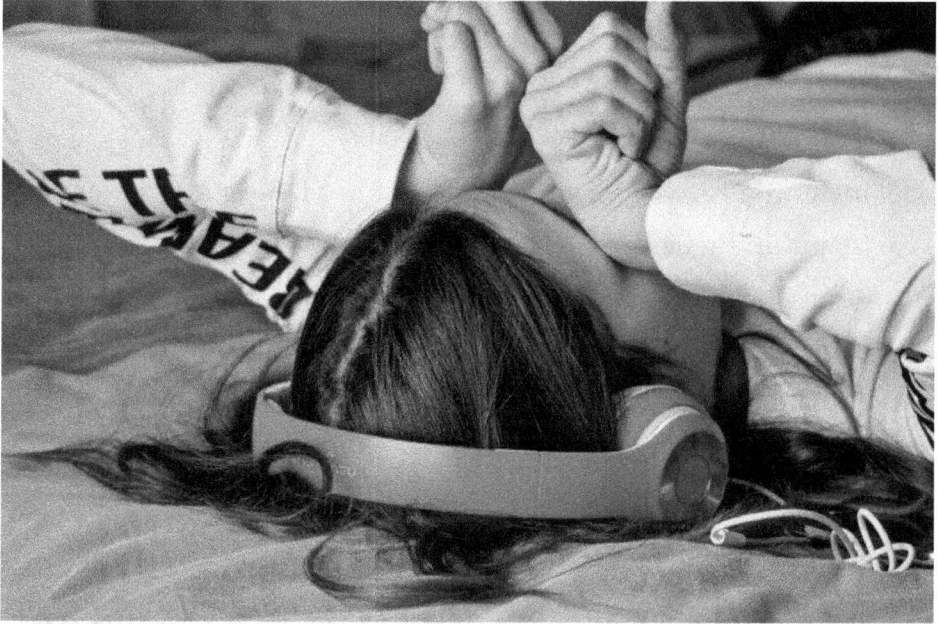

As you now have learned, there are various types and sub – categories of sleeping disorders. Sometimes it's genetic, sometimes it's a secondary factor to underlying conditions or illnesses whether physiological or mental, and sometimes it's also "man – made" due to poor sleeping habits and hygiene. Regardless, it's always important that you're aware of your condition, and you take the time to take care of your health by going to professional doctors, following their advice, and even doing your own research so that you can find alternative treatments. We hope this book helped you learn more about such disorders and guide you in getting a much better sleep. Quality sleep is your goal to achieve an active and healthy mind and body.

Various Types of Sleeping Disorders

Insomnia

Insomnia can be described as difficulty falling and maintaining asleep but for most people, perhaps it's simply another form of restlessness. Insomnia can be due to several causes including a mental disorder, medical condition, and constant exposure to drugs or other substances.

Classifications of Insomnia

- **Primary Insomnia:** This is a form of insomnia that is mostly attributed to psychological conditioning processes
- **Secondary Insomnia:** This is a form of insomnia that is attributed to psychiatric, external and medical causes.
- **Acute Insomnia:** Acute insomnia is usually caused by stress in life and emotional or physical discomforts.
- **Chronic Insomnia:** It is caused by various medical and external factors that can pose treatment challenges to both the doctors and patients.

Chronic Insomnia Types

- **Psychological Insomnia:** It is caused by a learned response that teaches one's body to not fall asleep when a person plans to fall asleep.

- **Idiopathic Insomnia:** It is perhaps one of the most detrimental cases because it can already occur at a very young age usually early childhood or even at the infancy stage, and progresses into adulthood.

- **Paradoxical Insomnia:** The termed 'paradoxical or misperception' is coined because this chronic form of insomnia is one where a patient complaints about experiencing insomnia without any actual evidence or symptom if the disorder.

- **Limit – Setting Disorder:** This is also known as Behavioral Insomnia, and it's a type of insomnia that occurs in infants and kids. Parents should also make sure that they practice sleeping hygiene on their children so that they can maintain this kind of habit and not have trouble sleeping.

- **Short – Term Insomnia Disorder:** External factors can cause short – term insomnia such as stress, anticipation, illness, excitement, changing schedules, time zones, pain due to loss of someone or something, reactions to certain medications, marital problems, financial, work or family problems etc.

Sleep – Related Breathing Disorders

Obstructive Sleep Apnea

It is one of the most common sleep – related breathing disorders next to insomnia. It is also quite dangerous and affects both adults and kids but the good news is that it can be easy to diagnosed and treated. This form of sleep disorder happens when the presence of hypopneas and obstructive apneas are repeated.

Central Sleep Apnea Syndrome

CSA is defined as repeated cessation of airflow in the lungs, and a concurrent cessation of respiratory effort.

Types of Central Sleep Apnea

- **Central Sleep Apnea with Cheyne – Stokes Breathing:** This is quite similar to what causes CSA but it is coupled with volume of breaths that forms a waning and waxing pattern which doctors see during the NREM or non – rapid eye movement.

- **Central Sleep Apnea Caused by Medical Disorders without Cheyne – Stokes Breathing:** Medical disorders like the so – called Degenerative Brainstem Lesions are known to contribute to central respiratory events wherein it becomes a secondary disorder.

- **Central Sleep Apnea Caused by High – Altitude Periodic Breathing:** This occurs when the central apneas and hypopneas of patients are raised whenever they reached an altitude of around 4,000 meters (12,000 feet).

Primary Central Sleep Apnea

In infants this occurs when babies have long respiratory events that are central or obstructive in nature, and something that lasts for about 20 seconds or so. Primary Central Sleep Apnea is also quite common in babies who are born premature. If this is the case, the newborn infants will usually require ventilator support.

Sleep – Related Hypoventilation Disorders

- **Obesity Hypoventilation Syndrome**
  This syndrome is also known as Hypercapnic Sleep Apnea; it is defined as hypoventilation that happens when the patients sleep.

- **Congenital Central Alveolar Hypoventilation Syndrome**
  This type of hypoventilation disorder is defined as the failure of the body's automatic central control of breathing

- **Late – Onset Central Hypoventilation with Hypothalamic Dysfunction**
  The symptoms can be diagnosed during the first few years of the child, and it includes obesity, lack of gene mutation (PHOX2B), and other sleep – related hypoventilation disorders.

- **Idiopathic Central Alveolar Hypoventilation**
  This type is characterized by the presence of alveolar ventilation that can result to sleep – related hypercapnia as well as hypoxemia in patients.

Isolated Symptoms

- **Snoring**
  Snoring is when a person creates audible vibrations in their upper lungs whenever they inhale or exhale during their sleep.

- **Catathrenia**
  Also known as sleep – related groaning, and this happens when there's a repeated groaning when a person exhales during their sleep (occurs in Rapid Eye Movement).

Central Disorders of Hypersomnolence

Narcolepsy Type I

It refers to the patient experiencing "sleep attacks" and its main cause is either a pathological or physiological abnormality. Symptoms include EDS (excessive daytime sleepiness), Rapid Eye Movement sleep phenomenon such as sleep paralysis and hypnogogic hallucinations as well as cataplexy.

- **Excessive Daytime Sleepiness**
  It's another common symptom usually seen in most narcoleptic patients. Patients are usually aware if there's an incoming "sleep attack" but they also can't help to unintentionally fall asleep at inappropriate times like in between conversations, while at work, or during sexual activity.

- **Cataplexy**
  It manifests in the body through feeling of mild muscle weakness to complete limb atonia that often results from the person falling. Narcoleptic patients experiencing cataplexy symptom usually drops whatever they are holding which can oftentimes be embarrassing for them or harmful to others.

- **Sleep Paralysis**
  This is defined as a partial to total paralysis of skeletal muscles once an individual wakes or at the onset of sleep.

Narcolepsy Type II

This is very similar to narcolepsy type I except for the fact that the cataplexy symptom is not present or being experienced by patients.

Idiopathic Hypersomnia

This is defined as the occurrence of refreshing naps, decreased sleep latency, and absence of cataplexy.

Kleine – Levin Syndrome

This is also known as Periodic Hypersomnolence or Recurrent Hypersomnia. It happens when a patient experiences series of episodes of excessive sleeping or hypersomnia.

Circadian Rhythm Sleep – Wake Disorders

- **Delayed Sleep – Wake Phase Disorder**
  This is described as a later sleep schedule than expected or desired by an individual.

- **Advanced Sleep – Wake Phase Disorder**
  This is quite the same with Delayed Sleep – Wake Phase Disorder but only this time a person falls asleep earlier that what one expects or desires.

- **Irregular Sleep – Wake Rhythm Disorder**
  It is described by having abnormal sleeping patterns and abnormal waking times.

- **Non – 24 Hour Sleep – Wake Rhythm Sleep Disorder**
  This is formerly referred to as "Free – Running Disorder." It is when the body's circadian rhythm is inconsistent with the 24 – hour clock.

- **Shift Work Disorder**
  Patients suffering from this disorder are those who are assigned in a so – called "graveyard shift" and as a result of their work shift, their circadian rhythm are disrupted which is why they experience EDS.

- **Jet Lag Disorder**

  This happens when an individual travels in more than 2 time zones.

Parasomnia

- **Confusional Arousals**

  This happens when an individual wakes up in a confused state.

- **Sleep Walking**

  Sleep walking occurs when certain behaviors such as sitting up, jumping, running, walking from bed happens during a slow wave sleep.

- **Sleep Terrors**

  This is a disorder that happens when one is awaken from the slow wave sleep while experiencing feelings of intense fear.

- **Sleep – Related Eating Disorder**

  This is when the person has repeated instances of eating or drinking during arousals while they're still sleeping.

- **Recurrent Isolated Sleep Paralysis**

  Sleep paralysis is usually a symptom of narcolepsy that happens when the person is unable to move during sleep (hypnagogic) or once they wake up (hypnopompic).

- **Nightmare Disorder**

  Nightmares among PTSD patients give them a hard time falling back to sleep because they are still traumatized about their dreams.

- **Exploding Head Syndrome**

  This is a sleep disorder where a person experiences an imagined loud noise or a sense of explosion while they are asleep or upon awakening.

- **Sleep – Related Hallucinations**

  Both hypnagogic and hypnopompic hallucinations happen in narcoleptic patients wherein they experience a sort of visual hallucination when they wake up or when they fall asleep.

- **Sleep Enuresis**

  This is also known as nocturnal enuresis. It happens when a person urinates several times while they sleep or the commonly known as bedwetting.

- **Sleep Talking**

  Sleep talking is quite common and can happen in any age while a person is sleeping.

Sleep – Related Movement Disorders

- **Restless Legs Syndrome**
- This is a kind of sleep – related movement disorder that's usually characterized by the body's urge to move in order to stop the odd sensations that usually can be felt in their legs.

- **Periodic Limb Movement Disorder**

  It is another common sleep disorder that is characterized when a patient involuntarily moves their legs or limbs while they are asleep.

- **Sleep – Related Leg Cramps**
  This kind of disorder is described as something intense because the patients usually feel a sudden burst of leg cramps while they sleep.

- **Sleep – Related Bruxism**
  Bruxism is the act of grinding one's teeth or the habit of jaw clenching while sleeping.

- **Sleep – Related Rhythmic Movement Disorder**
  It is described as a series of repetitive body movements while a person is sleeping or whenever the patient is experiencing some form of drowsiness.

- **Benign Sleep Myoclonus of Infancy**
  It is also known as limb jerks; it is simply the various body movements while an infant is sleeping.

- **Propriospinal Myoclonus at Sleep Onset**
  It happens when there are repetitive body movements in the neck, abdomen, and also the trunk part of the person's body during sleep.

Isolated Symptoms of Sleep – Related Movement Disorder

- **Excessive Fragmentary Myoclonus**
  This happens when the person is having frequent muscle twitches particularly in its fingers, mouth muscles, and toes upon awakening or while sleeping.

- **Hypnagogic Foot Tremor (HFT) and Alternating Muscle Activation (ALMA)**
  HFT is when the legs or foot movements have a rhythmic pattern once they fall asleep or during sleep. ALMA is relative similar with HFT but the only difference is that one leg usually follows the movement of the other leg.

- **Hypnic Jerks**
  Hypnic jerks is characterizes as a sudden muscle movement or jerk at the onset of sleep, and it's usually accompanies by feelings of falling, fear, or surprise.

Photo Credits

Page 1 Photo by user Free – Photos via Pixabay.com,

https://pixabay.com/en/sleep-bed-woman-bedroom-sleeping-1209288/

Page 7 Photo by user Jacob Steward via Flickr.com,

https://www.flickr.com/photos/jhstewart/5960469024/

Page 21 Photo by user Michelle Ress via Flickr.com,

https://www.flickr.com/photos/safoocat/1384616196/

Page 32 Photo by user Philips Communications via Flickr.com,

https://www.flickr.com/photos/philips_newscenter/10572460734/

Page 50 Photo by user Nadio via Flickr.com,

https://www.flickr.com/photos/nadio/408044508/

Page 60 Photo by user Rachel Tayse via Flickr.com,

https://www.flickr.com/photos/11921146@N03/6981949723/

Page 72 Photo by user Army Medicine via Flickr.com,

https://www.flickr.com/photos/armymedicine/11191238585/

Page 98 Photo by user Loren Kerns via Flickr.com,

https://www.flickr.com/photos/lorenkerns/4136759863/

Page 104 Photo by user sweetlouise via Pixabay.com,

https://pixabay.com/en/girl-young-woman-awakening-3231843/

References

Herbal Remedies and Sleep – Sleep Health Foundation
Organization

https://www.sleephealthfoundation.org.au/pdfs/HerbalRem
edies-0713.pdf

Management of Common Sleep Disorders by Dr. Kannan
Ramar, and Dr. Eric J. Olson via ThePAFP.org

http://thepafp.org/website/wp-
content/uploads/2017/09/Management-of-Common-Sleep-
disorders.pdf

Sleep Disorders – JB Publishing

http://samples.jbpub.com/9781284030273/Chapter2_Secure.p
df

**Sleep Disorders and Problems: Symptoms, Treatment,
and Self-Help** – HelpGuide.org

https://www.helpguide.org/articles/sleep/sleep-disorders-and-
problems.htm

Ten Common Sleep Disorders - Sleep Health Foundation
Organization

http://sleephealthfoundation.org.au/pdfs/facts/Common%20
Sleep%20Disorders.pdf

Treatment of Insomnia: An Alternative Approach by Anoja S. Attele, DDS, Jing-Tian Xie, MD, and Chun-Su Yuan, MD, PhD via SemanticsScholar.org

https://pdfs.semanticscholar.org/55e2/78c9ee7fffb71139e663c1295c07ad732628.pdf

Types of Sleep Disorders – WebMd.com

https://www.webmd.com/sleep-disorders/default.htm

Types of Sleep Disorders – News – Medical.net

https://www.news-medical.net/health/Types-of-sleep-disorders.aspx

Understanding Sleep Disorders – ClevelandClinic.org

https://my.clevelandclinic.org/ccf/media/Files/Neurological-Institute/sleep-disorders-center/understanding-sleep-disorders-treatment-guide.pdf

Understanding Sleep Disorders – American Academy of Neurology

http://patients.aan.com/globals/axon/assets/10026.pdf

What Are Sleep Disorders? – Healthline.com

https://www.healthline.com/health/sleep/disorders#types

www.ingramcontent.com/pod-product-compliance
Lightning Source LLC
Chambersburg PA
CBHW060908280326
41934CB00007B/1230